With the compliments of
BAYER AG, Research Department

W.-D. Busse B. Garthoff F. Seuter (Eds.)

Dihydropyridines

Progress in Pharmacology and Therapy

With 53 Figures and 6 Tables

Springer-Verlag
Berlin Heidelberg New York
London Paris Tokyo
Hong Kong Barcelona
Budapest

WOLF-DIETER BUSSE, Ph.D., Professor
International Research Pharma
BAYER AG
Aprather Weg 18 a
42096 Wuppertal
Germany

BERNWARD GARTHOFF, DVM
Cardiovascular and
Arteriosclerosis Research
BAYER AG
Aprather Weg 18 a
42096 Wuppertal
Germany

FRIEDEL SEUTER, Ph.D.
Coordination International Research
BAYER AG
Aprather Weg 18 a
42096 Wuppertal
Germany

ISBN-13: 978-3-540-57308-1 **e-ISBN-13: 978-3-642-95716-1**
DOI: 10.1007/ 978-3-642-95716-1

Typesetting: Best-set Typesetter Ltd., Hong Kong
27/3130/SPS-5 4 3 2 1 0 – Printed on acid-free paper

Preface

At the Pharmacology Workshop held in Wuppertal on December 11, 1992, Dr. Alexander Scriabine was honored for his contribution to drug development at our company.

Dr. Scriabine was the first pharmacologist to join Miles in West Haven, CT, in 1979. He established the Miles Institute for Preclinical Pharmacology, at the Yale campus, which was devoted to cardiovascular, metabolic and, later, CNS research. At that time Ca^{2+} antagonists were not yet available in the USA, but well established in Europe. At Bayer, Bossert and Vater discovered 1,4-dihydropyridines in the late 1960s, and Fleckenstein identified nifedipine as the most potent Ca^{2+} antagonist available at that time. This discovery led to the establishment of Ca^{2+} antagonists as leading cardiovascular drugs throughout the world and to the marketing of nifedipine as Adalat by Bayer. The main function of the Miles Institute for Preclinical Pharmacology was the introduction of Bayer Ca^{2+} antagonists to the American scientific community. Scriabine, in collaboration with Stanislav Kazda and Bernward Garthoff, contributed numerous publications on the pharmacology of Bayer Ca^{2+} antagonists, supported many collaborative studies with extramural investigators in the USA, and organized several international conferences on Ca^{2+} antagonists. These conferences contributed to the recognition of the importance of these drugs for the treatment of hypertension and coronary heart disease in North America.

Scriabine and his colleagues were also instrumental in the introduction of new technology for evaluating Ca^{2+} antagonists and other drugs. The first electrophysiology laboratory in the pharmaceutical industry was established at the Miles Institute for Preclinical Pharmacology by Charles Cohen and Richard McCarthy, and dihydropyridine receptors were characterized in a collaborative study between Ronald Janis of Miles and David Triggle of the State University of New York at Buffalo.

With the help of electrophysiological techniques, Richard McCarthy succeeded in demonstrating the effectiveness of Ca^{2+} antagonists at the single cell level. This technique was used to demonstrate direct neuronal action of nimodipine, a calcium antagonist discovered by Horst Meyer, Stanislav Kazda, and Friedrich Hoffmeister. Numerous pharmacological studies were undertaken at the Miles Institute for Preclinical Pharmacology, such as with BAY K 8644, a Ca^{2+} agonist, discovered by Matthias Schramm in Wuppertal.

This symposium reviews important milestones in the history of the development of 1,4-dihydropyridines as Ca^{2+} antagonists and includes presentations of the results of some recent collaborative extramural studies by American investigators.

Wuppertal, September 1993 WOLF-DIETER BUSSE

Contents

List of Authors

BEAN, B.P.
Department of Neurobiology, Harvard Medical School, 200 Longwood Avenue, Boston, MA 02115, USA

BECHEM, M.
BAYER AG, Cardiovascular and Arteriosclerosis Research, P.O. Box 10 17 09, 42096 Wuppertal, Germany

BUSSE, W.-D.
BAYER AG, International Research Pharma, P.O. Box 10 17 09, Aprather Weg 18a, 42096 Wuppertal, Germany

DISTERHOFT, J.F.
Department of Cell, Molecular, and Structural Biology, Northwestern University Medical School, 303 East Chicago Avenue, Chicago, IL 60611-3008, USA

ELLER, A.
BAYER AG, Cardiovascular and Arteriosclerosis Research, P.O. Box 10 17 09, 42096 Wuppertal, Germany

FRANZ, J.K.
BAYER AG, Cardiovascular and Arteriosclerosis Research, P.O. Box 10 17 09, 42096 Wuppertal, Germany

GARTHOFF, B.
BAYER AG, Cardiovascular and Arteriosclerosis Research, P.O. Box 10 17 09, 42096 Wuppertal, Germany

GOLDMANN, S.
BAYER AG, Pharma Research, Chemistry Department, P.O. Box 10 17 09, 42096 Wuppertal, Germany

GROSS, R.
BAYER AG, Cardiovascular and Arteriosclerosis Research, P.O. Box 10 17 09, 42096 Wuppertal, Germany

HEBISCH, S.
BAYER AG, Cardiovascular and Arteriosclerosis Research, P.O. Box 10 17 09, 42096 Wuppertal, Germany

HÜTTER, J.
BAYER AG, Cardiovascular and Arteriosclerosis Research, P.O. Box 10 17 09, 42096 Wuppertal, Germany

KAZDA, S.
BAYER AG, Cardiovascular and Arteriosclerosis Research, P.O. Box 10 17 09, 42096 Wuppertal, Germany

KOWALSKA, M.
Department of Cell, Molecular, and Structural Biology, Northwestern University Medical School, 303 East Chicago Avenue, Chicago, IL 60611-3008, USA

MINTZ, I.M.
Department of Neurobiology, Harvard Medical School, 200 Longwood Avenue, Boston, MA 02115, USA

MOYER JR, J.R.
Department of Cell, Molecular, and Structural Biology, Northwestern University Medical School, 303 East Chicago Avenue, Chicago, IL 60611-3008, USA

RAE, P.
BAYER AG, Cardiovascular and Arteriosclerosis Research, P.O. Box 10 17 09, 42096 Wuppertal, Germany
and
Miles Research Center, 400 Morgan Lane, West Haven, CT 06516, USA

ROUNDING, P.
BAYER AG, Cardiovascular and Arteriosclerosis Research, P.O. Box 10 17 09, 42096 Wuppertal, Germany

SCHRAMM, M.
BAYER AG, Cardiovascular and Arteriosclerosis Research, P.O. Box 10 17 09, 42096 Wuppertal, Germany

SCRIABINE, A.
Miles Institute for Preclinical Pharmacology, 400 Morgan Lane, West Haven, CT 06516, USA

SPREYER, P.
BAYER AG, Cardiovascular and Arteriosclerosis Research, P.O. Box 10 17 09, 42096 Wuppertal, Germany

STAAY, F.J. VAN DER
BAYER-Tropon Institute for Neurobiology, Troponwerke, Berliner Str. 156, 51063 Cologne, Germany

STOLTEFUSS, J.
BAYER AG, Pharma Research, Chemistry Department, P.O. Box 10 17 09, 42096 Wuppertal, Germany

THOMPSON, L.T.
Department of Cell, Molecular, and Structural Biology, Northwestern University Medical School, Chicago, 303 East Chicago Avenue, IL 60611-3008, USA

TRABER, J.
BAYER-Tropon Institute for Neurobiology, Troponwerke, Berliner Str. 156, 51063 Cologne, Germany

TRIGGLE, D.J.
School of Pharmacy, State University of New York, Buffalo, NY 14260, USA

UNTERBECK, A.
BAYER AG, Cardiovascular and Arteriosclerosis Research, P.O. Box 10 17 09, 42096 Wuppertal, Germany
and
Miles Research Center, 400 Morgan Lane, West Haven, CT 06516, USA

VRY, J. DE
BAYER-Tropon Institute for Neurobiology, Troponwerke, Berliner Str. 156, 51063 Cologne, Germany

WATTS, J.A.
Department of Biology, University of North Carolina at Charlotte, Charlotte, NC 28223, USA

Twenty Years of Dihydropyridines*

S. Kazda

The first comprehensive publication describing the pharmacological properties of a dihydropyridine (DHP) prototype appeared 20 years ago in several papers of the January 1972 issue of Drug Research (Arzneimittelforschung). Since then, several thousands of scientific papers on DHPs have been published. Nevertheless, the results of the extensive pharmacological investigations of nifedipine, performed by Bayer scientists and reported in the introductory article of the January issue of *Arzneimittelforschung* by Vater et al. [1] remain valid as pars pro toto for the DHP group of calcium antagonists. Only the overall interpretation of these data, which appeared in the discussion in that first DHP paper, should be read in a historical context, based on the knowledge of 1972.

Coronary Heart Disease

The goal of the "father of nifedipine," Dr. Wulf Vater, was to find a coronary dilating drug for the treatment of ischemic heart disease. With this in mind, Vater introduced techniques to measure oxygen content in the coronary sinus blood of experimental animals. These techniques indirectly permitted estimation of the coronary dilating effects of compounds under study (Fig. 1).

At that time, two drugs (carbocromen and dipyridamole) were known to dilate coronary arteries, and Vater used them as reference compounds in his experiments. The therapeutic value of these drugs became increasingly burdened by the "steal effect" they had on the diseased heart. Since both are generally potent dilators of the intramural resistance vessels, their effect in the diseased heart is more pronounced in healthy areas and results in a redistribution of the blood supply at the expense of the ischemic region ("steal"). A worsening of chest pain in some patients was observed, and this led to a general rejection by cardiologists of pharmacogenic coronary dilation as a therapeutic principle.

---

* Dedicated to Dr. Wulf Vater on the occasion of his 75th birthday.

Institute for Cardiovascular and Arteriosclerosis Research, Bayer AG, P.O. Box 10 17 09, Wuppertal, Germany 42096

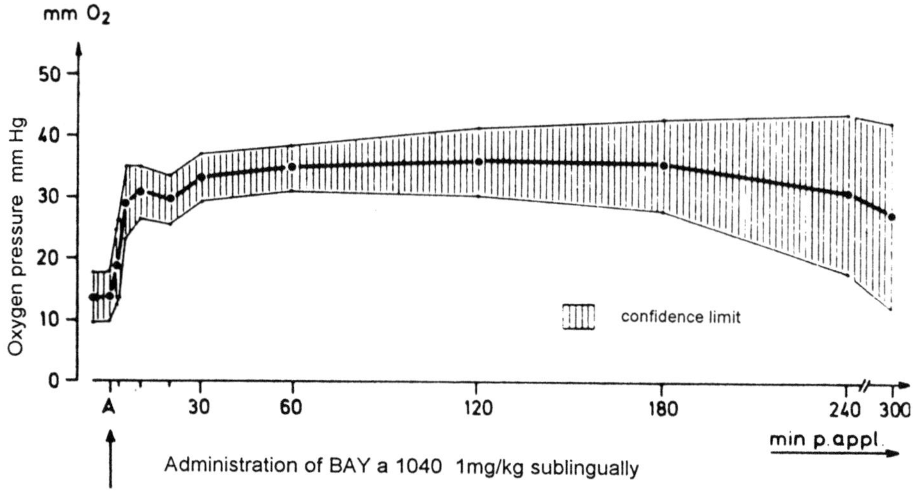

Fig. 1. Increase in the partial pressure of oxygen in dog coronary sinus after sublingual administration of nifedipine (1 mg/kg). (From [1])

However, the pharmacological profile of nifedipine differed from that of the existing "coronary vasodilators." It became obvious that the coronary dilation effect in response to different drugs is not always the same. In contrast to steal producing drugs such as carbocromen and dipyridamole, nifedipine also dilates the large extramural branches of the coronary arteries with their collaterals and not only the intramural resistance arterioles. This effect of nifedipine improves blood flow in the ischemic regions of the heart, and the steal effect is replaced by a kind of "Robin Hood" effect, i.e., taking from the rich and giving to the poor.

So, Vater's dream of finding new and better coronary vasodilators became a reality, requiring further investigation at the Institute of Pharmacology at Bayer. Under the leadership of Professor Kroneberg, the pharmacologists Hoffmeister, Kaller, Meng, Oberdorf, Puls, Schloßmann, and Stoepel carried out a pharmacological analysis of the effects of this new compound. Soon it became clear that enhancement of the oxygen supply to the heart was not the only effect of the 1,4-dihydropyridines. More detailed investigations revealed two other cardiovascular actions which were at least as important as the increase in coronary oxygen observed during the initial test, but these were not deemed particularly desirable in coronary patients. First, the decrease in blood pressure was known from early experiments with high doses in anesthetized dogs. Now, using conscious hypertensive animals, it was also present after the therapeutic dose and was rather strong. How could this be tolerated by angina patients who also have hypertension? This question occupied Bayer scientists for a long time and will thus be discussed here extensively. Later I shall also explain which additional investigations contributed to reformulation of the question such that this "side effect" could be utilized for the treatment of hypertension.

The second undesirable effect was exactly the same as that enabling Fleckenstein to discover "calcium antagonism" with prenylamine and verapamil, namely, the pronounced negative inotropic action on the heart. The extensive published discussion of this effect [1], which resulted in creation of a new term, "regulated inotropy," appeared nearly acrobatic in its argumentation, but the validity of the conclusions was later confirmed by hemodynamic investigations and therapeutical trials.

Further experiments, mainly those of Taira [2] and Henry [3], demonstrated that nifedipine's calcium antagonism differs from that of verapamil, especially regarding the ratio of the coronary dilating and cardiac inhibiting effects. In contrast to verapamil, the negative inotropic effect of nifedipine is much smaller than its vasodilatory effect, and nifedipine does not have a depressant effect on cardiac nodes. Moreover, the negative inotropic effect on the myocardium obviously does not contribute to therapeutic efficacy in patients with coronary heart disease, whereas in vivo myocardial contractility is increased after nifedipine due to sympathetic counterregulation of the decreased peripheral resistance. The oxygen consumption of the diseased heart may actually be reduced not by a cardiodepressive effect but by a reduced afterload due to the peripheral vasodilation.

But this was not known in 1972. Rather, Fleckenstein still postulated an "action of nifedipine on cardiac energy metabolism" [4] as a therapeutic principle in ischemic heart disease: nifedipine, like other calcium antagonists

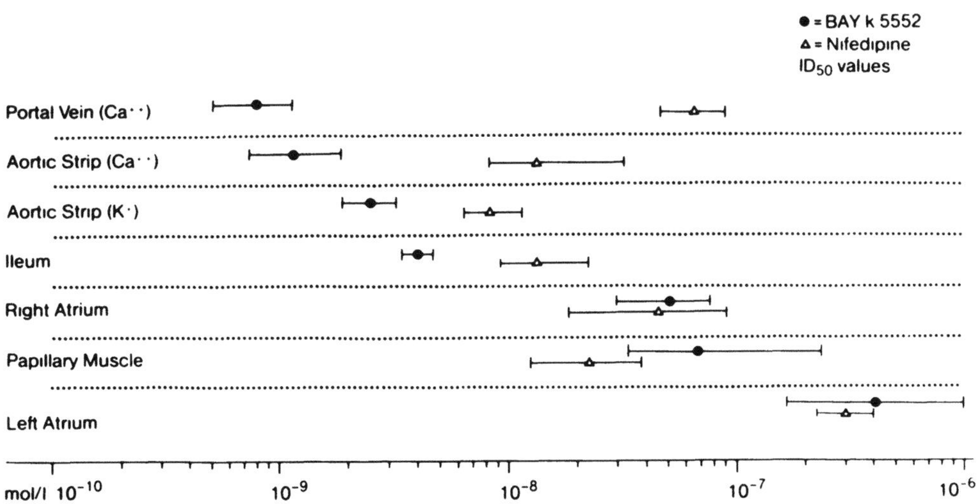

Fig. 2. Inhibitory effects of nisoldipine on isolated smooth muscle and cardiac preparations in vitro: a comparison with nifedipine. (From [5])

known at that time, restricts calcium-dependent adenosine triphosphate consumption, contractile energy expenditure, and the oxygen requirement in active heart muscle.

The uncertainty regarding the clinical relevance of the negative inotropic effect of nifedipine stimulated further research at Bayer, specifically, looking for DHP derivatives with a more favorable ratio of vascular and cardiac "calcium antagonism." The keystone of the research was BAY K 5552, nisoldipine [5], a pioneering example of "vascular selectivity" among DHP derivatives (Fig. 2), a claim later repeatedly declared for other DHP compounds of competitor companies. Moreover, the vasorelaxing effect of nisoldipine is not uniformly localized in all vascular beds. Even compared to nifedipine, nisoldipine more potently relaxes the spasm of coronary arteries than that of peripheral arteries in vitro [6].

Less negative inotropy and more coronary selectivity together with prolonged duration of action are the prominent properties of nisoldipine, favoring its use in the treatment of ischemic heart disease at present.

Hypertension

The DHP calcium antagonists are currently the drugs of choice in the first step treatment of essential hypertension. This is not a surprise since arterial vessels are the target of their calcium antagonistic effect, resulting in decreased elevated peripheral resistance. However, it was not until the early 1980s that the antihypertensive effect has been promoted by Bayer pharmacologists and accepted by clinicians. Calcium antagonists were like a "Sleeping Beauty" in hypertension, mainly because of another dilemma arising in early pharmacological investigations. In short-term standard experiments, nifedipine reduced diuresis and renal excretion of sodium, presumably by reduction of renal filtration due to the decrease in blood pressure [1]. In that sense, DHPs have properties in common with other vasodilators in hypertension, making additional diuretic medication necessary.

Our experiments with long-term treatment in hypertensive rats raised substantial doubts as to whether these standard experiments disclosed the real effects of DHPs on the kidney. In 1982, we published results showing that "The antihypertensive effect of calcium antagonists differs from that of vasodilators" [7], mainly because of the different effects on the kidney. Whereas hydralazine and minoxidil produced sodium retention with a subsequent increase in body fluids, nifedipine and other DHPs enhanced sodium excretion. While common vasodilators aggravated heart hypertrophy, despite a lowering of the pressure in hypertension, DHPs caused a regression of cardiomegaly in our experiments, presumably by reducing both volume load and blood pressure at the same time. At present, the beneficial effect of long-term treatment with DHPs on the size and performance of the hypertensive heart has been established.

Even in acute experiments, a single substitution of tap water for oral induction of diuresis by saline unmasked a clear-cut natriuretic and diuretic effect of DHPs [8]. These effects are solely due to the inhibition of tubular reabsorption of sodium, nitrendipine being more potent than nifedipine [9]. The natriuretic effect of nifedipine had already been observed in 1972 in the clinical trial carried out by Klütsch et al. and described in Drug Research (Arzneimittelforschung) together with a series of publications on nifedipine [10]. For nearly a decade the effect went unnoticed. It was unusual and therefore improbable (or even impossible), since according to textbooks pharmacological vasodilation had to reduce sodium excretion.

We now know that the renal effect of DHP calcium antagonists is rather complex. In normotensives they increase natriuresis by inhibiting sodium reabsorption in the proximal tubule, probably by inhibiting sodium-calcium exchange. In hypertensives, at least during the initial phase of therapy, the glomerular filtration rate also increases [11]. It is now established that long-term treatment with nifedipine or nitrendipine leads to a long-term change in sodium balance. This effect certainly contributes to the antihypertensive efficacy of DHPs.

Vascular Protection

Our investigations on the kidneys presented us with another surprise. We obtained interesting strains of rats which had varying sensitivity to dietary salt load, the Dahl rats. One substrain, the sensitive (S) substrain, rapidly develops malignant hypertension on a high salt diet, whereas the other, resistant (R), substrain, tolerates salt without any symptoms. In the S rats, the salt load resulted not only in hypertension but also in early vascular damage, arteriolosclerosis localized mainly in the kidney (Fig. 3) and mesenterium, and in premature death. Treatment with nifedipine prevented hypertension and vascular lesions completely [12]. The latter should not necessarily be surprising if one considers that the lesions were the consequence of hypertension and not the toxic effect of salt. Dr. Luckhaus, our pathologist, however, was surprised when I and Dr. Garthoff sent him the kidneys from S rats which had first received nifedipine at the malignant stage, when some of them were in a moribund state. With nifedipine treatment they all recovered, and Dr. Luckhaus found very few lesions in the kidneys; there were mainly residues from preexisting changes and clear signs of healing, regeneration of the elastic lamina, reendothelization, etc. [13]. Skeptical as pathologists are, he suspected that we had sent him the wrong samples. We repeated the experiments several times, also using other DHPs, and we got the same results. The high blood pressure was partially lowered, but remained within the hypertensive range, but in the kidneys and mesenteric arteries of the rats treated with DHPs the lesions were minimal and in the process of healing (Fig. 4).

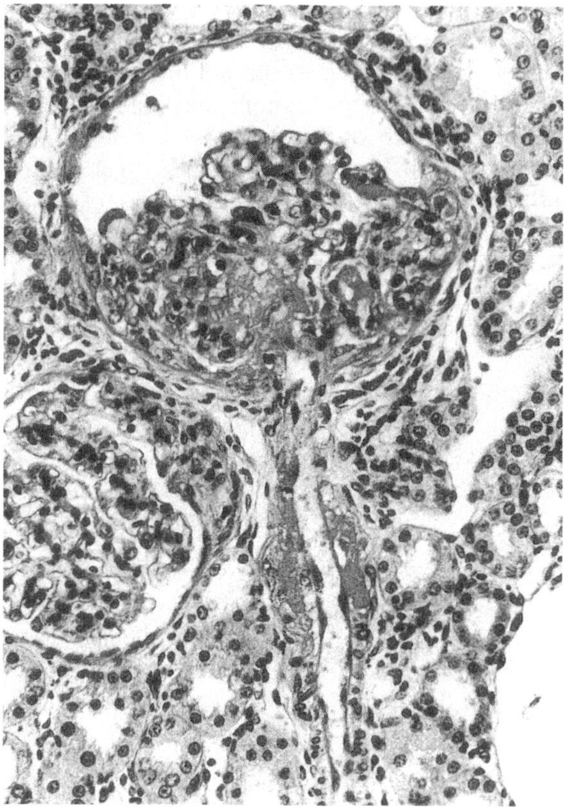

Fig. 3. Necrotizing vasculopathy in the kidney of salt-loaded Dahl S rats. Fibrinoid impregnation of the afferent arteriole and glomerular collapse. (From [13])

We suggested that nifedipine prevented progressive tissue damage and induced its repair by not, or not only, decreasing the pressue, but also probably as a result of its direct tissue protective effect. In addition to high pressure, some other factors are obviously responsible for the tissue damage in hypertensive disease. One hypothesis includes calcium overload as one of these factors. In later experiments with other rat strains (stroke-prone, spontaneously hypertensive rats, SHR) and with another DHP derivative, nimodipine, which has only a weak effect on peripheral vessels, we confirmed this hypothesis and extended its validity to other pathological states such as experimental stroke [14].

Fleckenstein, in his early work with high doses of vitamin D3, demonstrated the destructive power of excessive calcium entry into the vascular wall. It turned out that mitochondria and contractile structures rapidly disintegrated as soon as the intracellular concentration of calcium ions surpassed the tolerable limit. "Calcium is the killer," shouted Fleckenstein

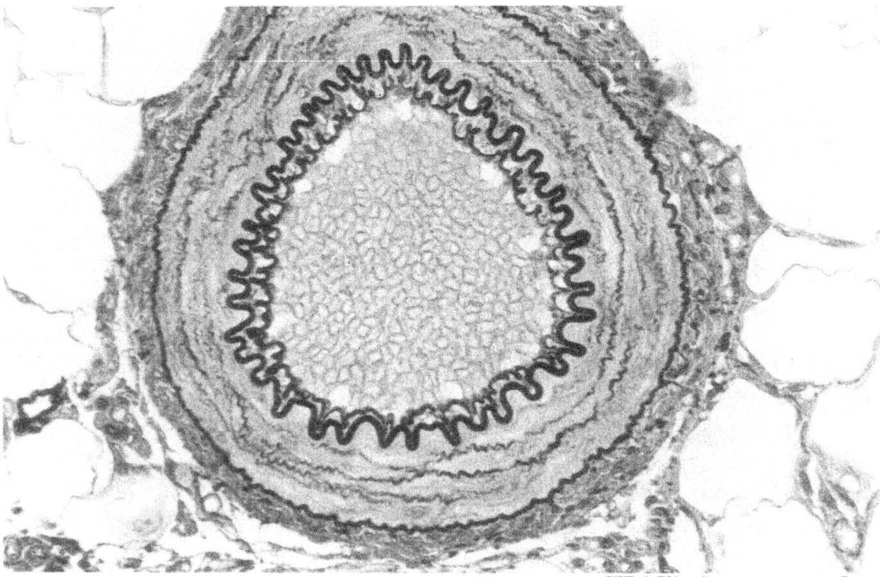

Fig. 4. Histological features of healing of malignant hypertensive arteriopathy in the mesentery of a Dahl S rat after 6 week treatment with nifedipine. Intimal fibrin resorption has taken place, supporting reendothelization. An additional elastic lamina has formed on the luminal side of the original internal elastic lamina. (From [13])

during a passionate discussion with his incredulous opponents at an international conference in 1972 in Freiburg.

Our experiments with Dahl rats and later with stroke-prone SHR demonstrated that severe vascular damage which occurs spontaneously or is accelerated by dietary salt in clinically relevant models of cardiovascular diseases has a similar pathogenesis as the vitamin D3 poisoning in Fleckenstein's rats. We demonstrated that this calcium overload may also be prevented or even repaired by using nifedipine and its analogues. We speculated that some calcium-regulating system is activated in advanced or accelerated hypertension which induces excessive calcium entry into the vascular wall via a DHP-sensitive pathway. We demonstrated that an excess of some parathyroid-derived substance may be involved. Calcium antagonists blocking the deleterious calcium overload maintain cellular integrity and appear to be life-saving drugs [14].

In experimental medicine, our finding of the tissue protective effect of calcium antagonists in Dahl rats is well accepted, especially as Fleckenstein confirmed it years later and published these results, with acknowledge of our priority, in several review articles (e.g., [15]). The clinical validity of our finding on the tissue protective effect of DHPs in Dahl rats is now being tested in human studies. Especially with nitrendipine, renal protection was demonstrated in hypertensive but also in other patients suffering from ischemic or toxic renal damage.

Atherosclerosis

Another calcium-dependent vascular wall disease, atherosclerosis, which has an extremely high incidence and few therapeutic possibilities, is at present the focus of clinical DHP research. Atherosclerosis has traditionally been regarded as the result of disorders in lipid metabolism. The plasma levels of cholesterol fractions are generally high in patients, and the impregnation of diseased vessel regions by cholesterol is regarded as an early step in the pathogenesis of the disease. The recent idea, that calcium ions are involved in the early stage of atherosclerotic plaque formation, has many sponsors [16].

Fleckenstein investigated the composition of the walls of thousands of vessels from forensic autopsies in humans 1–90 years of age. The most impressive finding was the steady age-dependent rise in the aortic calcium content, being 50–100 times higher in old people than in children. Interestingly, the aortic cholesterol content begins to increase much later, and in the oldest group investigated it reached values which were only six times higher than those measured in the youngest age group. This and the above-cited experimental findings on the detrimental role of calcium in the vascular wall allowed Fleckenstein to postulate that calcium – and not cholesterol – is the key factor in atherogenesis, a possibility which had been neglected by scientists until now [15].

A seemingly opposite view, by Henry, ultimately led to similar assumptions being made about the early involvement of calcium in atherogenesis. Henry worked with isolated coronary arteries in vitro and found that adding cholesterol to the bath induced contractions by stimulating calcium influx [17]. These contractions could be inhibited by nifedipine. Extrapolation into in vivo conditions was obvious. The excess plasma cholesterol opens up vascular pathways for the entry of calcium ions, which increase the tone and also damage the vascular wall. Both calcium and cholesterol participate in the formation of atherosclerotic plaques. Consequently, Henry performed a critical experiment which opened up new horizons for the future of nifedipine. He induced atherosclerosis in rabbits fed a high cholesterol diet, a procedure which has long been used in this research field. The rabbits developed plaques in the aortae, and the walls of nonatherosclerotic aortic regions were rich in both cholesterol and calcium. In rabbits receiving prolonged nifedipine treatment in addition to a high cholesterol diet, the appearance of atherosclerotic plaques was largely prevented. The calcium and cholesterol content also remained normal in the healthy regions, despite the fact that the high plasma concentration of cholesterol was not affected by nifedipine [18].

It is difficult to decide which of these – calcium or cholesterol – is the chicken and which the egg. However, the final result is fascinating: inhibition of calcium entry by nifedipine prevents the pathological event, i.e., atherosclerotic damage of the vessel wall. This experiment initiated a lively discussion with several pros and contras, as is usual with unusual findings. It also excited clinicians, especially those with open minds to new ideas. Lichtlen, an experienced researcher in the area of calcium antagonists, organized a large multicenter study of patients with atherosclerosis. After 3 years of accurately controlled observations, long-term treatment with nifedipine was found to have no effect on already existing plaques in coronary arteries, but dramatically inhibited progression of the disease. The number and size of new atherosclerotic plaques was much smaller in patients treated with nifedipine [19].

Meanwhile a similar positive influence on atherogenesis has been confirmed by several other clinical studies, so that the vision of a revolutionary impact of DHPs on cardiovascular morbidity seems justified, as atherosclerosis is currently the most important disabling and lethal vascular disease of our time.

Calcium Channels

The DHPs, nifedipine, nitrendipine, nisoldipine, and nimodipine and numerous successors from competitors, became commercially successful drugs substantially improving the therapeutic armamentarium of cardiovascular medicine and neurology. Moreover, as substances with a well defined mechanism and high specifity of action, DHPs also became tools in biological, physiological, and pathophysiological research on the role of calcium ions and their cellular regulation. Thanks to the DHPs, the structural features and the molecular pharmacology of the calcium channel in the cell membrane could be explored. The existence of a slow channel for calcium ions as a special transmembrane carrier system in heart muscle had been proposed many years ago, based on electrophysiological phenomena [20]. The importance of such slow calcium channels in the excitation-contraction coupling in cardiac and smooth muscle was underlined by the identification of specific calcium channel blocking agents, the "calcium antagonists," typified by verapamil, nifedipine and diltiazem, as described by Fleckenstein [21].

Two fundamental discoveries of Bayer pharmacologists regarding DHPs enabled further identification of the precise structure and function of the calcium channel. In 1981, Bellemann, in cooperation with Glossmann and his group at Gießen, used tritiated nitrendipine to discover a stereospecific high-affinity binding site on cardiac membranes. Bellemann et al. concluded that "this site may represent the structure of a supposed calcium channel where the potent 1,4 dihydropyridine calcium antagonists are proposed to bind and act" [22]. Schramm et al., in 1983, found that small modifications

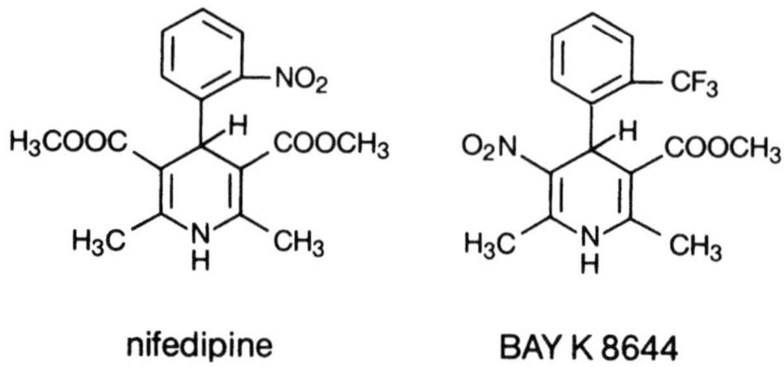

Fig. 5. Formulas of nifedipine and BAY K 8644

to the nifedipine molecule produced other DHP derivatives, e.g., BAY K 8644 (Fig. 5), with effects diametrically opposite to those of the calcium antagonists: cardiac contractility is stimulated and smooth muscle is contracted. These effects are competitively antagonized by nifedipine but not by verapamil or diltiazem. This observation provided "the first evidence that there exist some sites in or near the calcium channel which bind DHP derivatives, and that occupation of these sites may either increase ("calcium agonists", for example, BAY K 8644) or decrease ("calcium antagonists", for example, nifedipine) the transmembrane calcium influx into the cell" [23].

BAY K 8644 and the related calcium agonists discovered by Schramm were not useful as therapeutic agents since they also constricted coronary arteries. Further concentrated effort was necessary in both chemical and pharmacological research to find cardioselective derivatives which could be developed as new cardiotonic drugs. Results of this work are summarized by Groß (this volume).

The discoveries of both stereospecific DHP binding sites and specific ligands as competitive agonists initiated an explosion of biochemical, molecular biological, electrophysiological, and pharmacological research, resulting in thousands of scientific publications. The excellent results in elucidating the structure and function of the calcium channel and the implications of these findings were summarized in a Bayer Centenary Symposium at Stresa 1988 [24].

The existence of a DHP receptor within the calcium channel and the potency and selectivity of DHP ligands as exogenous calcium channel modulators suggest that there may be some endogenous factor which physiologically operates or modulates calcium channel function. Its discovery may be anticipated as a logical consequence of the intensive and fruitful research with DHPs over the last 20 years. It certainly will open up new possibilities in the search for new specifically tailored therapeutics.

References

1. Vater W, Kroneberg G, Hoffmeister F, Kaller H, Meng K, Oberdorf A, Puls W, Schloßmann K, Stoepel K (1972) Zur Pharmakologie von 4-(2'-Nitrophenyl)-2,6-dimethyl-1,4-dihydropyridin-3,5-dicarbonsäuredimethylester (Nifedipin, BAY a 1040). Arzneimittelforschung 22:1–170
2. Taira N, Motomura S, Narimatsu A, Ijima T (1975) Experimental pharmacological investigations of effects of nifedipine on atriventricular conduction in comparison with those of other coronary vasodilators. In: Lochner W, Braasch W, Kroneberg G (eds) New therapy of ischemic heart disease. 2nd international Adalat symposium. Springer, Berlin Heidelberg New York, pp 40–48
3. Henry PD (1980) Comparative pharmacology of calcium antagonists: nifedipine, verapamil and diltiazem. Am J Cardiol 46:1047–1058
4. Fleckenstein A, Grün G, Byon KY, Döring HJ, Tritthart H (1975) The basic Ca antagonistic actions of nifedipine on cardiac energy metabolism and vascular smooth muscle tone. In: Hashimoto K, Kimura E, Kobayashi T (eds) New therapy of ischemic heart disease. 1st international nifedipine "Adalat" symposium: University of Tokyo Press, pp 31–44
5. Kazda S, Garthoff B, Meyer H, Schloßmann K, Stoepel K, Towart R, Vater W, Wehinger E (1980) Pharmacology of a new calcium antagonistic compound, isobutyl methyl 1,4-dihydro-2,6-dimethyl-4-(2-nitrophenyl)-3,5-pyridinedicarboxylate (Nisoldipine, BAY K 5552). Arzneimittelforschung 30 (II, 12):2144–2162
6. Kazda S (1991) Inhibitory effects of nisoldipine on serotonin and potassium induced contractions of porcine coronary and femoral arteries. Arzneimittelforschung 41:204–207
7. Kazda S, Garthoff B, Thomas G (1982) Antihypertensive effect of calcium antagonists in rats differs from that of vasodilators. Clin Sci 63:363s–365s
8. Garthoff B, Knorr A, Thomas G, Kazda S (1982) Nitrendipine increases sodium excretion in acutely saline loaded rats. Biochem Pharmacol 31:3015–3016
9. Johns ES, Mauritius J (1987) The renal actions of nitrendipine and its influence on the renal regulation of calcium and sodium reabsorption in the rat. J Cardiovasc Pharmacol 9 [Suppl 1]:S49–S56
10. Klütsch K, Schmidt P, Grosswendt J (1972) Der Einfluß von BAY a 1040 auf die Nierenfunktion des Hypertonikers. Arzneimittelforschung 22:377–380
11. Kazda S, Hirth C, Stasch JP (1988) Diuretic effect of nitrendipine contributes to its antihypertensive efficacy. A review. J Cardiovasc Pharmacol 12 [Suppl 4]: S1–S5
12. Kazda S, Garthoff B, Dycka J, Iwai J (1982) Prevention of malignant hypertension in salt loaded "S" Dahl rats with the calcium antagonist nifedipine. Clin Exp Hypertens A4:115–121
13. Luckhaus G, Nash G, Garthoff B, Kazda S, Feller W (1985) Healing of malignant hypertensive arteriopathy in Dahl rats by nifedipine. Arzneimittelforschung 35:115–121
14. Kazda S, Grunt M, Hirth C, Preis W, Stasch JP (1987) Calcium antagonism and protection of tissues from calcium damage. J Hypertens 5 [Suppl 4]:S37–S42
15. Fleckenstein A, Frey M, Zorn J, Fleckenstein-Grün G (1990) Calcium, a neglected key factor in hypertension and arteriosclerosis: experimental vasoprotection with calcium antagonists or ACE-inhibitors. In: Laragh JH, Bramer BM

(eds) Hypertension: pathophysiology, diagnosis and management. Raven, New York, pp 471–510
16. Kazda S (1991) The story of nifedipine. In: Lichtlen PR, Reale A (eds) Adalat. Springer, Berlin Heidelberg New York, pp 9–26
17. Henry PD, Witztum JL, Yokoyama M (1978) Vasoconstrictor effect of low density lipoprotein on canine coronary artery. Circulation 58 [Suppl II]:297
18. Henry PD, Bentley KI (1981) Suppression of atherogenesis in cholesterol fed rabbit treated with nifedipine. J Clin Invest 68:1366–1369
19. Lichtlen PR, Hugenholtz PG, Rafflenbeul W, Hecker H, Jost S, Deckers JW (1990) Retardation of angiographic regression of coronary artery disease by nifedipine. Lancet 335:3–7
20. Reuter H, Beeler GW (1969) Calcium current and activation of contraction in ventricular myocardial fibres. Science 162:399–401
21. Fleckenstein A (1970/71) Specific inhibitors and promotors of calcium action in the excitation-contraction coupling of heart muscle and their role in the production or prevention of myocardial lesions. In: Harris P, Opie L (eds) Calcium and the heart. Academic, London, pp 135–188
22. Bellemann P, Ferry D, Lübbecke F, Glossmann H (1981) [^{3}H]-Nitrendipine, a potent calcium antagonist, binds with high affinity to cardiac membranes. Arzneimittelforschung 31:2064–2067
23. Schramm M, Thomas G, Towart R, Franckowiak G (1983) Novel dihydropyridines with positive inotropic action through activation of Ca^{++} channels. Nature 303:535–537
24. Morad M, Nayler W, Kazda S, Schramm M (1988) The calcium channel: structure, function and implications. Springer, Berlin Heidelberg New York

1,4-Dihydropyridines and the 1,4-Dihydropyridine Receptor

D.J. Triggle

Introduction

The 1,4-dihydropyridine nifedipine is a first-generation drug of major significance in the treatment of cardiovascular disorders including hypertension, peripheral vascular disorders and angina in its several forms. Nifedipine is one of a chemically and pharmacologically heterogeneous group of drugs that includes also verapamil and diltiazem and which owe their cardiovascular properties to a specific interaction with one cellular route of calcium entry – the L-type voltage-gated calcium channel (reviewed in Fleckenstein 1983; Janis et al. 1987).

The discovery of the group of drugs collectively referred to as the calcium antagonists is linked closely to an understanding of the roles and control of cellular calcium metabolism (reviewed in Campbell 1983). Calcium plays dual roles in cellular function. Under physiological conditions of temporal and spatial control calcium is a central player in the paradigm of stimulus-response coupling. Under pathological conditions of uncontrolled mobilization calcium mediates cell death and destruction (Cheung et al. 1986). Drugs that control aberrant calcium mobilization processes may, therefore, be expected to be therapeutically usefull agents for cardiovascular,
neuronal and other cellular disorders. However, efforts to control calcium mobilization must recognize the plurality (and redundancy) of calcium control processes and the consequent multiplicity of potential drug binding sites (Campbell 1983; Janis et al. 1987).

The history of the discovery of 1,4-dihydropyridines has been reviewed by their discoverers (Bossert and Vater 1989). The 1,4-dihydropyridine nucleus has proved not only to be a potent pharmacophore for calcium channel antagonists, but this same structure has also generated potent calcium channel activators. Since many of the interactions of 1,4-dihydropyridines with calcium channels are powerfully voltage-dependent, minor changes in structure and cellular conditions can produce both quantitative and qualitative changes in pharmacologic activities. Additionally the 1,4-dihydropyridine nucleus yields ligands active at other classes of ion channels and membrane

School of Pharmacy State University of New York, Buffalo, NY 14260, USA

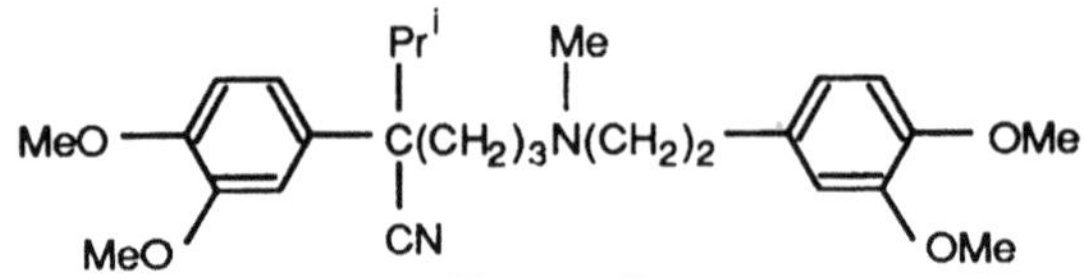

Verapamil

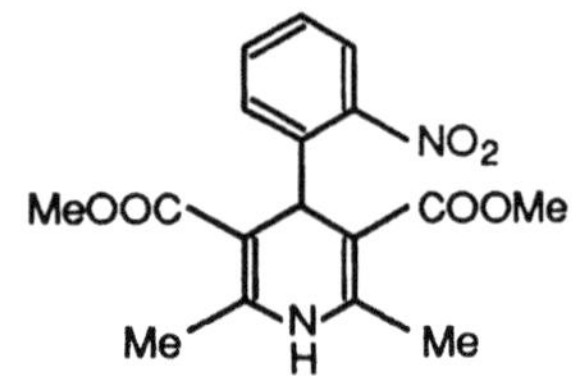

Nifedipine

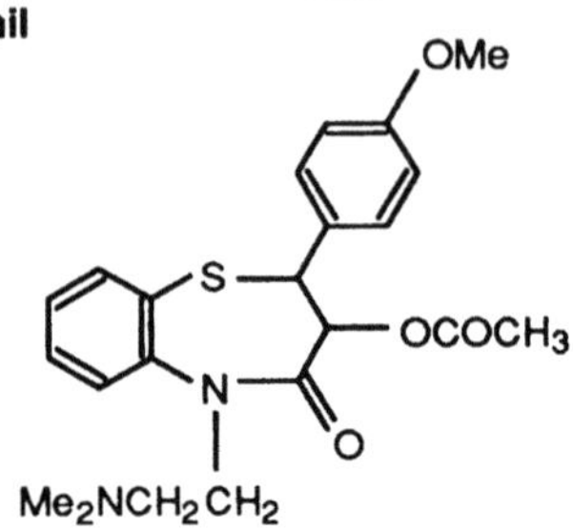

Diltiazem

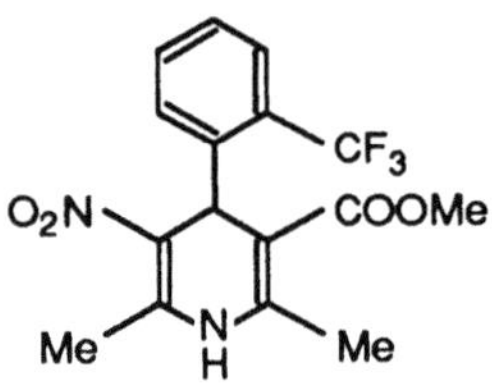

Bay k 8644

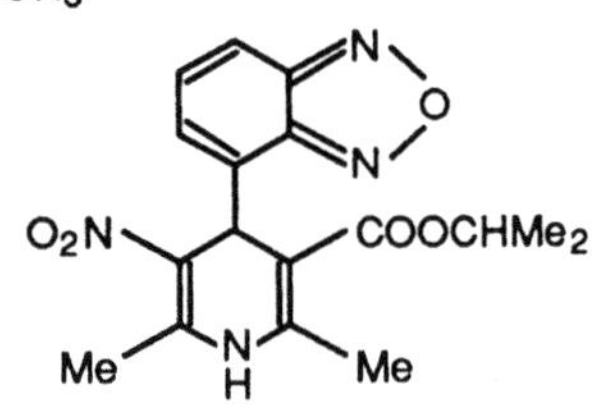

PN 202 791

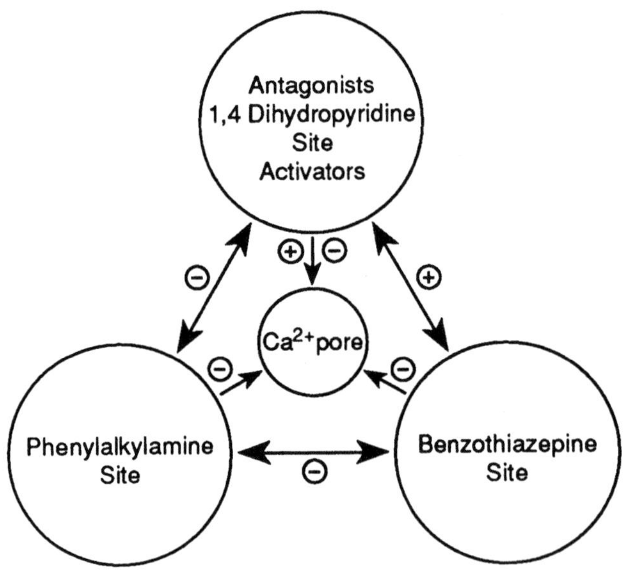

Fig. 1. The organization of the principal drug binding sites at the L-type voltage-gated calcium channel

receptors (Rampe and Triggle 1993). Thus 1,4-dihydropyridines may represent privileged structures capable of interacting with a variety of transmembrane proteins.

Calcium Antagonist Binding Sites

Evidence drawn primarily from radioligand binding studies indicates, consistent with the observed pharmacologic and chemical heterogeneity, that the calcium channel antagonists interact at discrete binding sites associated with a major protein of the L-type voltage-gated channel (Janis et al. 1987; Glossmann and Striessnig 1988). Figure 1 depicts drug binding sites linked both to the functional machinery of the channel and to each other by heterotropic allosteric interactions. From these interactions are derived the existing and potential therapeutic roles of these drugs (Table 1).

Table 1. Uses and potential uses of calcium channel antagonists

Cardiovascular	*Nonvascular smooth muscle*
Angina	Achalasia
Arrhythmias (selected)	Asthma
Atherosclerosis	Dysmenorrhea
Cardioplegia	Eclampsia
Cerebral ischemia, focal	Esophageal spasm
Cerebral ischemia, global	Intestinal hypermotility
Congestive heart failure	Obstructive lung disease
Hypertension	Premature labor
Hypertrophic cardiomyopathy	Urinary incontinence
Migraine	
Myocardial infarction	
Peripheral vascular diseases	
Subarachnoid hemorrhage	
Other	
Aldosteronism	
Antimalarial drug resistance	
Cancer chemotherapy (multiple drug resistance)	
Epilepsy	
Glaucoma	
Manic syndrome	
Motion sickness	
Spinal cord injury	
Tinnitus	
Tourette's disorder	
Vertigo	

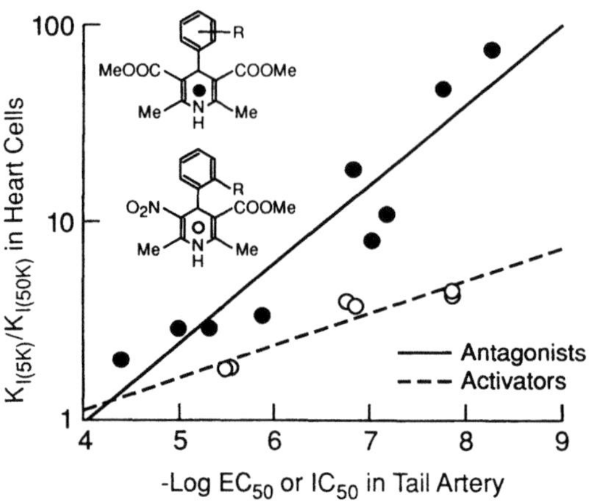

Fig. 2. Voltage-dependent binding of 1,4-dihydropyridine antagonists (nonchiral) and activators [*S*-enantiomers] to rat ventricular myocytes. The ratio $K_{I(5K)}/K_{I(50)K}$ is an index of voltage-dependent binding in myocytes and the EC_{50} and IC_{50} values are indices of potency in vascular smooth muscle. (From Zheng et al. 1992)

Several questions may be raised concerning the representation of Fig. 2. There likely exist more than three drug binding sites associated with the L-type channel: indeed, recent evidence suggests that there may exist as many as six or more discrete drug binding sites associated with this channel (reviewed in Rampe and Triggle 1990, 1993). However, therapeutic exploitation of these additional sites is still in its infancy. Additionally, the existence of potent antagonist and activator ligands for this effector suggests that endogenous ligands may exist for which the existing drugs are mere synthetic surrogates (Triggle 1988). However, only candidate species exist thus far for the endogenous ligand.

The Calcium Channel as a Pharmacologic Receptor

The voltage-gated calcium channel may be regarded as a pharmacologic receptor characterized by both electrophysiologic and pharmacologic criteria (Table 2). As pharmacologic receptors these channels will be expected to possess the following general characteristics:

1. The presence of drug binding sites with defined structure-activity relationships, including stereoselectivity, for both activators and antagonists. Endogenous ligands may exist.
2. The drug binding sites will be coupled to the permeation and gating machinery of the channel.
3. The channel may be coupled to regulatory guanine nucleotide (G) binding proteins.

Table 2. Classification of voltage-gated calcium channels

Property	L	T	N	P
Conductance, pS	25	8	12–20	10–12
Activation threshold	High	Low	High	Moderate
Inactivation rate	Slow	Fast	Moderate	Rapid
Permeation	$Ba^{2+} > Ca^{2+}$	$Ba^{2+} = Ca^{2+}$	$Ba^{2+} > Ca^{2+}$	$Ba^{2+} > Ca^{2+}$
Function	E-coupling: cardiovascular system, smooth muscle, endocrine cells and some neurons	Cardiac SA node: spiking, repetitive spike activity in neurons and endocrine cells	Neuronal only: neurotransmitter release	Neuronal only(?): neurotransmitter release
Pharmacologic sensitivity: 1,4-dihydropyridines (activators/antagonists), phenylalkylamines benzothiazepines	Sensitive	Insensitive	Insensitive	Insensitive
ω-Conotoxin	Sensitive (some)?	Insensitive	Sensitive	Insensitive
Octanol, amiloride	Insensitive	Sensitive	Insensitive	?
Funnel web spider toxin and ω-Agatoxin	Insensitive	Insensitive	Insensitive	Sensitive

4. The channels will be regulated by homologous and heterologous influences.
5. Channel number and function may be altered during disease states and thus contribute to the pathology of the disease.

These expectations have, with the exception of the discovery of an endogenous ligand (Triggle 1988), been generally realized (Janis et al. 1987; Janis and Triggle 1991).

The 1,4-Dihydropyridine Receptor

The 1,4-dihydropyridine structure has attracted particular attention because it has generated the most potent of the calcium channel antagonists, because it exhibits both antagonist and activator properties and because structural change, including stereochemistry, is accompanied by major changes in biologic activity. A number of important questions may be raised:

1. What are the structural requirements for activation and antagonism?
2. Do activators and antagonists interact at the same site or at separate sites?
3. Where is the binding site for the 1,4-dihydropyridines?
4. What is the basis for the selectivity of action of the 1,4-dihydropyridines?
5. Is the 1,4-dihydropyridine site regulated?

These issues have been discussed in a number of recent reviews (Catterall and Striessnig 1992; Janis et al. 1987; Janis and Triggle 1991; Triggle et al. 1989).

Structure-Activity Relationships

Although the structure-activity relationships of 1,4-dihydropyridines have been well discussed in the literature (reviewed in Bossert and Vater 1989; Goldmann and Stoltefuss 1991; Janis et al. 1987; Manger et al. 1992; Triggle et al. 1989), it is increasingly clear that these relationships must be discussed in terms of the voltage-dependent interactions of the 1,4-dihydropyridines (Triggle 1989). Unfortunately, only limited studies are available to apply to structure-activity considerations.

In a series of antagonists (nonchiral) and activators (*S*-enantiomers) the influence of membrane potential upon activity in cardiomyocytes reveals significant differences (Zheng et al. 1992). Confirming previous isolated observations (Ferrante et al. 1989; Kokubun et al. 1986; Wei et al. 1989) antagonist and activator binding were potential-dependent and potential-independent, respectively (Fig. 2). This is consistent with major differences between activator and antagonist binding modes. Furthermore, the extent of voltage-dependence of antagonist binding increased with increasing potency of the antagonist. These data suggest the possibility that the future design of

1,4-dihydropyridines should include as one further molecular variable the influence of membrane potential. Almost certainly the tissue selectivity patterns observed with the 1,4-dihydropyridines have their origins significantly based in this relationship between structure and voltage-dependence of interactions.

The Regulation of 1,4-Dihydropyridine Receptors

Previous work has described the homologous and heterologous regulation of voltage-gated calcium channels (reviewed in Ferrante and Triggle 1990). Quite generally chronic channel occupancy or activation produces complementary changes in receptor number and function. Thus, chronic depolarization of PC12 cells (DeLorme et al. 1988) and chick retinal neurons (Ferrante et al. 1991) down-regulates channel number and function. It is of interest that L-type channels in cardiac cells, although demonstrating very similar pharmacology, are not similarly regulated by depolarization. The ability to regulate channel number and function may be a general property of neuronal cells since we have observed it also in rat cerebellar granule cells, PC12 cells and GH3 and GH4C1 cells (Bangalore et al. 1992). Of particular interest is that the depolarization-induced down-regulation has two components. One component is produced by chronic activation (hours to days) and is slowly reversible while the other component is produced by periods of depolarization extending from 5 to 120 min (Table 3) and is rapidly reversible. This process occurs during protocols for radioligand binding in intact cells (Table 3) and may well be of physiological significance offering considerable plasticity to neuronal calcium channels under conditions of use and disuse.

Calcium channels are also regulated during aging and several workers have proposed critical and central roles for changes in neuronal calcium homeostasis during the aging process (Gibson and Peterson 1987; Landfield 1987; Peterson et al. 1989). Recent reports that nimodipine may be clinically beneficial in dementias of aging (Ban et al. 1990; Tollefson 1990) and experimentally beneficial in memory and performance paradigms in aging

Table 3. Voltage-dependent binding of [^{3}H]PN 200 110 to rat cerebellar cells

Ligand	K^+ (mM)	K^D ($10^{-10}M$)	B_{max} (fmoles/mg)
PN 200 110	5.8	3.75	364.2
	50	0.25	70.6
R (+)-nimodipine	5.8	9.4	—
R (+)-nimodipine	50	1.3	—
S (−)-nimodipine	5.8	7.6	—
S (−)-nimodipine	50	0.9	—

animals focus new attention on the L-type channel of the brain (Deyo et al. 1989a,b). In the Fischer 344 rat significant changes are noted in the numbers of both L- and N-type channels with aging (Bangalore et al. 1992). These reductions in channel density are region-specific and age-dependent and are well marked in the cortex and striatum: they likely contribute to the cognitive and behavioral deficits seen in these animals upon aging.

1,4-Dihydropyridines as Privileged Structures

Although the 1,4-dihydropyridines are widely viewed as ligands specific for L-type channels, they exhibit also significant pharmacologic activities at other receptors including both ion channels and G-protein-coupled receptors (Rampe and Triggle 1993).

T-type calcium channel currents in adrenal glomerulosa cells and GH3 cells are blocked by nitrendipine and felodipine, respectively, with K_D values for the inactivated state of approximately $10^{-7}\,M$ (Cohen et al. 1988, 1992). In atrial cells, however, felodipine is significantly more active, with a

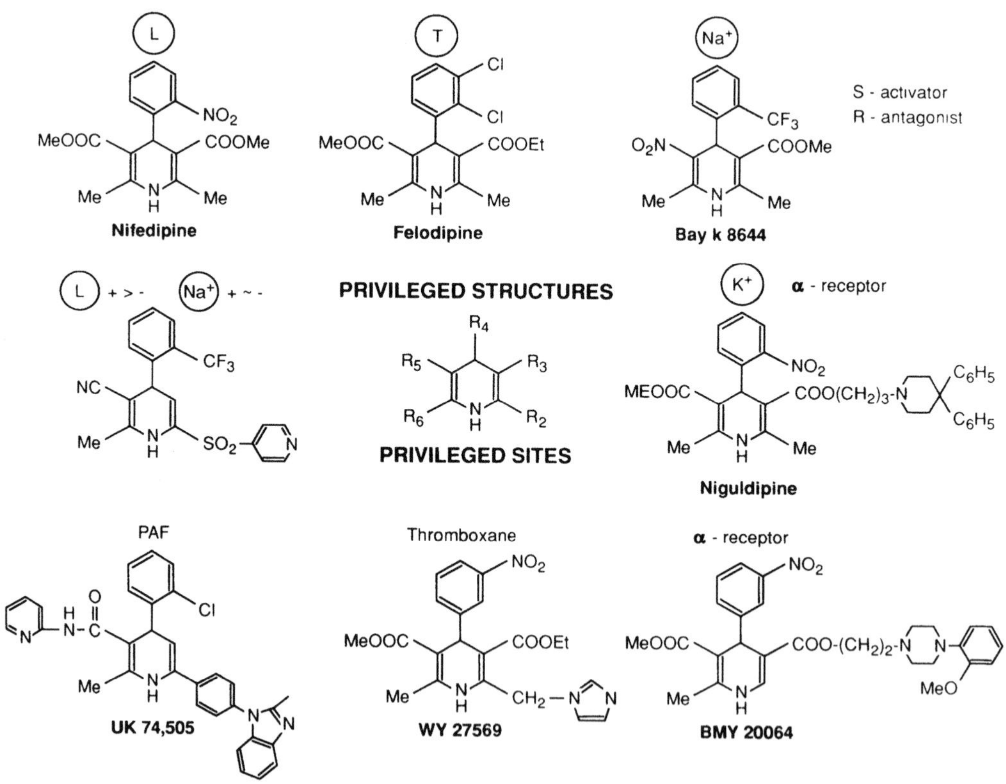

Fig. 3. 1,4-Dihydropyridines as privileged structures

K_D value for the inactivated state of $1.3 \times 10^{-8} M$ compared to $4 \times 10^{-10} M$ for the L-type channel (Cohen et al. 1992). Isradipine and (−) *R* 202 791 show similar potency differences between T- and L-type channels (Cohen et al. 1992).

1,4-Dihydropyridines also serve as modulators of other types of ion channels. Thus, nitrendipine blocks Na^+ channels with a K_D value of $3 \times 10^{-6} M$ and the *S* and *R* enantiomers of Bay K 8644 are activator and antagonist, respectively, at the Na^+ channel (Yatani and Brown 1985; Yatani et al. 1988). Niguldipine is an effective activator of Ca^{2+}-activated K^+ channels (Klockner et al. 1989) and nicardipine and Bay K 8644 block transient voltage-dependent K^+ currents in cardiomyocytes at micromolar concentrations (Gotoh et al. 1991).

Finally, the 1,4-dihydropyridine nucleus can serve as a pharmacophore for other membrane receptor and effector classes. A number of hybrid molecules can serve as dual Ca^{2+} channel-adrenoceptor, -thromboxane synthetase, -NO donor molecules (Rampe and Triggle 1993). However, particular attention is due molecules such as UK 74505 that serve as potent and selective platelet-activating factor (PAF) receptor antagonists with no actions at Ca^{2+} channels (Cooper et al. 1992). The 1,4-dihydropyridine structure may thus constitute a privileged species that interacts at privileged sites in membrane proteins.

Summary

The 1,4-dihydropyridines have proved to be extremely valuable therapeutic agents in the cardiovascular area and to offer considerable promise for development into neuronal areas of application. Simultaneously, the use of 1,4-dihydropyridines to identify specific receptors associated with a major class of voltage-gated calcium channel has been of major importance to the understanding of channel function and structure. That 1,4-dihydropyridines may constitute privileged structures interacting at privileged sites is likely to ensure their continued molecular and therapeutic prominence.

Acknowledgments Preparation of this work was supported by grants from NIH (HL 16003, GM 42850). Additional support from Miles, Inc. (West Haven, CT) and Fisons Inc. (Rochester, NY) is gratefully acknowledged.

References

Ban TA et al. (1990) Nimodipine in treatment of old age dementias. Prog Neuropsychopharmacol Biol Psychiatry 14:525–551

Bangalore R, Ferrante J, Hawthorn M, Zheng W, Rutledge A, Gopalakrishnan M, Triggle DJ (1992) The regulation of neuronal calcium channels. In: Proceedings

of the 5th international symposium on calcium antagonists, Houston, TX 1991. Plenum, New York (in press)
Bossert F, Vater W (1989) 1,4-Dihydropyridines as a basis for developing new drugs. Med Res Rev 9:291–324
Campbell AK (1983) Intracellular calcium: its universal role as regulator. Wiley, New York
Catterall WA, Striessnig J (1992) Receptor sites for Ca^{2+} channel antagonists. Trends Pharmacol Sci 13:256–262
Cheung JY, Bonventre JV, Malis CD, Leaf A (1986) Calcium and ischemic injury. N Engl J Med 314:1670–1676
Cohen CJ, McCarthy RT, Barnett PQ, Rasmussen H (1988) Ca channels in adrenal glomerulosa cells: K^+ and angiotensin II increase T-type Ca channel current. Proc Natl Acad Sci USA 85:2412–2416
Cohen CJ, Spires S, van Skiver D (1992) Block of T-type Ca channels in guinea pig atrial cells by antiarrhythmic agents and Ca channel antagonists. J Gen Physiol 100:703–728
Cooper K, Fray MJ, Parry MJ, Richardson K, Steele J (1992) 1,4-Dihydropyridines as antagonists of platelet activating factor. I. Synthesis and structure-activity relationships of 2-(4-heterocyclyl) phenyl derivatives. J Med Chem 35:3115–3129
DeLorme EM, Rabe CS, McGee R (1988) Regulation of the number of voltage-dependent Ca^{2+} channels in PC12 cells by chronic changes in membrane potential. J Pharmacol Ther 244:838–843
Deyo RA, Straube KT, Disterhoft JF (1989a) Nimodipine facilitates associative learning in aging rabbits. Science 243:809–811
Deyo RA, Straube KT, Moyer JR, Disterhoft JF (1989b) Nimodipine ameliorates age-related changes in open-field behavior of the rabbit. Exp Aging Res 15: 169–175
Ferrante J, Triggle DJ (1990) Drug- and voltage-induced regulation of voltage-dependent calcium channels. Pharmacol Rev 42:29–44
Ferrante J, Luchowski E, Rutledge A, Triggle DJ (1989) Binding of a 1,4-dihydropyridine calcium channel activator, (−) S Bay K 8644, to cardiac preparations. Biochem Biophys Res Commun 158:149–154
Ferrante J, Rutledge A, Triggle DJ (1991) The effects of chronic depolarization on L-type 1,4-dihydropyridine-sensitive voltage-dependent calcium channels in chick neural retina and rat cardiac cells. Can J Physiol Pharmacol 69:914–920
Fleckenstein A (1983) Calcium antagonism in heart and smooth muscle: experimental facts and therapeutic prospects. Wiley, New York
Gibson G, Peterson C (1987) Calcium and the aging nervous system. Neurobiol Aging 8:329–343
Glossmann H, Striessnig J (1988) Calcium channels. Vitam Horm 44:155–328
Goldmann S, Stoltefuss J (1991) 1,4-Dihydropyridines: effects of chirality and conformation on the calcium antagonist and calcium agonist activities. Ang Chem [Int Ed Eng] 30:559–578
Gotoh Y, Imaizumi Y, Watanabe M, Shibata EF, Clark RB, Giles WR (1991) Inhibition of transient outward K^+ current by DHP Ca antagonists and agonists in rabbit cardiac myocytes. Am J Physiol 260:H1737–1742
Janis RA, Triggle DJ (1991) Drugs acting on calcium channels. In: Hurwitz L, Partridge DL, Leach JK (eds) Calcium channels: their properties, functions, regulation and clinical relevance. CRC Press, Boca Raton, pp 195–249

Janis RA, Silver P, Triggle DJ (1987) Drug action and cellular calcium regulation. Adv Drug Res 16:309–591

Klockner U, Trieschmann Y, Isenberg G (1989) Pharmacological modulation of calcium and potassium channels in isolated vascular smooth muscle cells. Arz neimittel forschung 39:120–126

Kokubun S, Prod'hom B, Becker C, Porzig H, Reuter H (1986) Studies on Ca-channels in intact cardiac cells: voltage-dependent effects and cooperative interactions of dihydropyridine enantiomers. Mol Pharmacol 30:571–584

Landfield PW (1987) "Increased calcium current" hypothesis of aging. Neurobiol Aging 8:346–347

Manger PP, Coburn RA, Solo AJ, Triggle DJ, Rothe H (1992) QSAR, diagnostic statistics and molecular modelling of 1,4-dihydropyridine calcium antagonists: a difficult road ahead. Drug Des Discov 8:273–289

Peterson C, Ratan R, Shelanski M, Goldmann (1989) Changes in calcium homeostasis during aging and Alzheimers's disease. Ann N Y Acad Sci 568:262–270

Rampe D, Triggle DJ (1990) New ligands for L-type Ca^{2+} channels. Trends Pharmacol Sci 11:112–115

Rampe D, Triggle DJ (1993) New synthetic ligands for L-type calcium channels. Prog Drug Res 40:191–238

Tollefson GD (1990) Short-term effects of the calcium channel blocker nimodipine in the treatment of primary degenerative dementia. Biol Psychiatry 27:1133–1142

Triggle DJ (1988) Endogenous ligands: myths and realities. In: Morad M, Nayler WE, Kazda S, Schramm M (eds) The calcium channel: structure, function and implications. Springer, Berlin Heidelberg New York, pp 549–562

Triggle DJ (1989) Structure-function correlations of 1,4-dihydropyridine calcium channel antagonists and activators. In: Hondeghem LM (ed) Molecular and cellular mechanisms of antiarrhythmic agents. Futura, Mt Kiscoe, pp 269–292

Triggle DJ, Langs DA, Janis RA (1989) Ca^{2+} channel ligands: structure-function relationships of the 1,4-dihydropyridines. Med Res Rev 9:123–180

Wei X-Y, Rutledge A, Triggle DJ (1989) Voltage-dependent binding of 1,4-dihydropyridine Ca^{2+} channel antagonists and activators in cultured neonatal rat ventricular myocytes. Mol Pharmacol 35:541–552

Yatani A, Brown AM (1985) The calcium channel blocker nitrendipine blocks sodium channels in neonatal rat cardiomyocytes. Circ Res 56:868–875

Yatani A, Kunze DL, Brown AM (1988) Effects of dihydropyridine calcium channel modulators on cardiac sodium channels. Am J Physiol 254:H140–147

Wei X-Y, Rutledge A, Triggle DJ (1989) Voltage-dependent binding of 1,4-dihydropyridines in cultured neonatal rat ventricular myocytes. Mol Pharmacol 35:541–552

Zheng W, Stoltefuss J, Goldmann S, Triggle DJ (1992) Pharmacologic and radioligand binding studies of 1,4-dihydropyridines in rat cardiac and vascular preparations: stereoselectivity and voltage-dependence of antagonist and activator interactions. Mol Pharmacol 41:535–541

1,4-Dihydropyridines: Effects of Chirality and Conformation on Their Activity*

S. Goldmann and J. Stoltefuß

Introduction

About 10 years ago, minor changes in the structure of calcium antagonistic 1,4-dihydropyridines (Fig. 1, item 1) were found to lead to derivatives with diametrically opposed pharmacological effects (Fig. 1). The replacement of one ester group by the nitro group converts calcium antagonists to calcium agonists, in this case to BAY K 8644 (Fig. 1, item 2) the best investigated example in this series [1]. After separation of the enantiomers of BAY K 8644 it was discovered that only the (−)-S-enantiomer exhibits the calcium agonistic effects, while the other antipode is still a classical antagonist [2].

If you remove the right ester and replace it with hydrogen, the agonist *S*-2 changes into a weak antagonist, *R*-3. If you repeat the procedure with the other enantiomer, the weak antagonist *R*-2 will change into a weak agonist *S*-3 (see Fig. 1) [3].

In contrast the replacement of the nitro group with hydrogen changes the strong agonistic enantiomer *S*-2 into a weak agonist *S*-4 (Fig. 1) but it is still an agonist. The replacement of the nitro group of the antagonist *R*-2 by hydrogen has no significant change of activity (*R*-4) [4]. The change of the 2-CF_3-phenyl group to the 3-nitrophenyl group is not essential for activity, but in this case we know the absolute configuration of the antipodes of 4. Here, we would like to develop a simple model which explains the antagonistic or agonistic activities of these enantiomers and other derivatives.

The questions we have to answer are: (1) Which are the bioactive conformations of antagonists and agonists and (2) What is the important, the essential, difference between them?

* Dedicated to Professor R.W. Hoffmann on the occasion of his 60th birthday.
Bayer AG, Pharma Research, Chemistry Department, P.O. Box 10 17 09, 42096 Wuppertal, Germany.

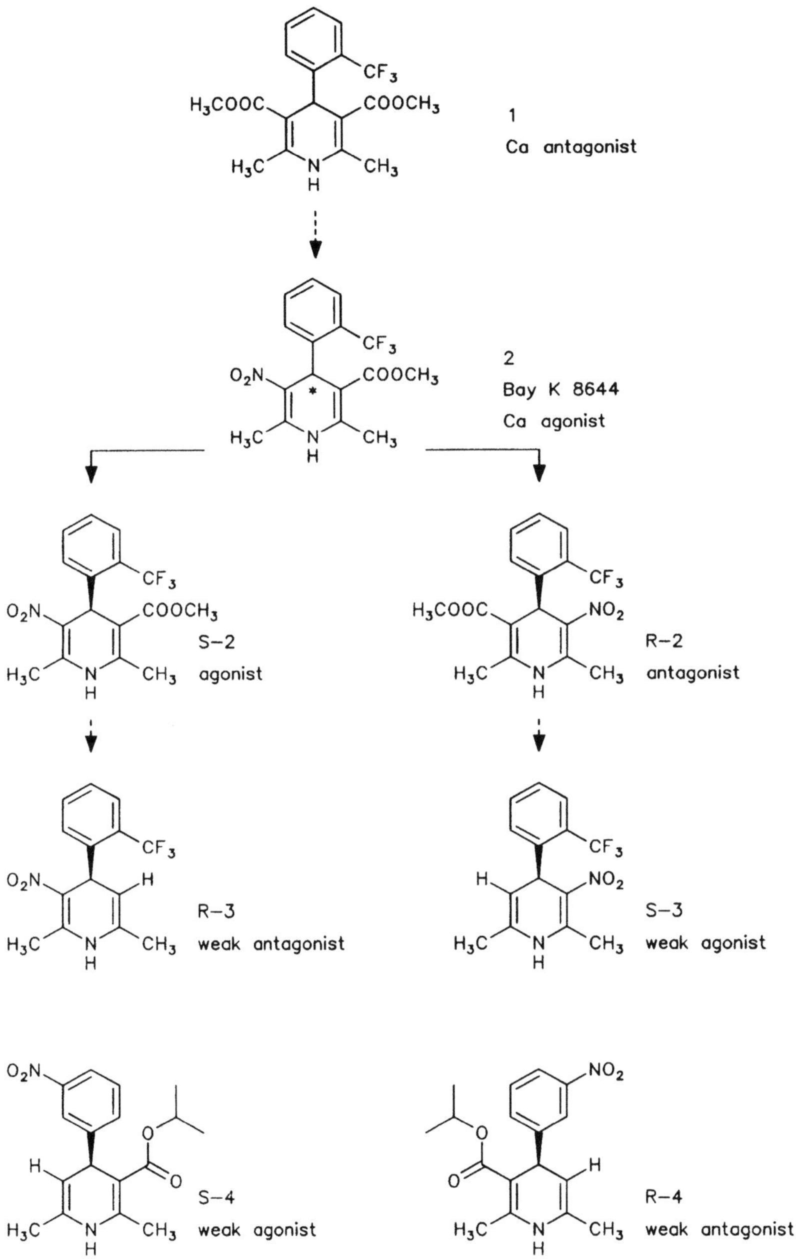

Fig. 1. Antipodes with opposed pharmacological activity

Conformation of the 1,4-Dihydropyridine Ring and Position of the 4-Aryl Substituent

In 1,4-dihydropyridines the ring is not planar but a flat boat (Fig. 2). The 4-phenyl substituent may occupy a pseudoaxial position (Fig. 2, item 5) or it may be equatorial (Fig. 2, item 6). Interconversion between the two forms is possible by inversion of the dihydropyridine ring. Further rotamers can be visualized if the 4-aryl ring is substituted in the ortho or meta position (X#H). The group X may then either be on the same side as the hydrogen (Fig. 2, item 5) or, following rotation of the phenyl ring, it may be above the dihydropyridine ring (Fig. 2, item 7). These rotamers are also conceivable if the aryl substituent is in the pseudo equatorial position (see Fig. 2, items 6 and 8).

Many X-ray structures indicate that the conformation shown in Fig. 2, item 5, is the most important conformation in crystal [5]. Some investigations with "fixed rotamers" indicate that this conformation is also important in solution at the receptor [5–8].

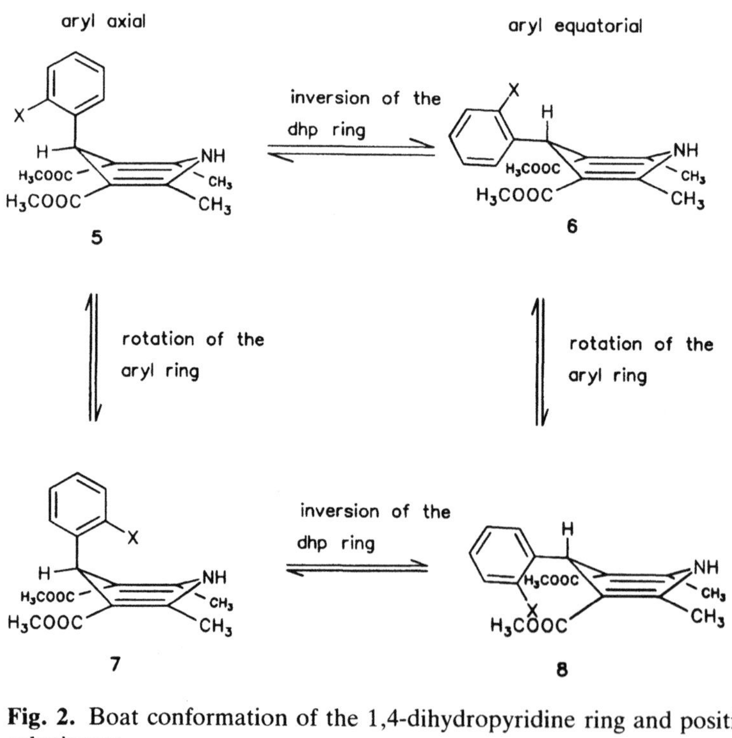

Fig. 2. Boat conformation of the 1,4-dihydropyridine ring and position of the 4-aryl substituent

Influence of the Ester Groups on the Pharmacological Effect

The ester groups are of crucial importance to the pharmacological effect. Not only does variation of the ester groups lead to quantitative changes in activity, but replacement of an ester groups by other groups (i.e., nitro or H) changes antagonists to agonists.

A method that has been adopted by Triggle et al. [9] to distinguish clearly between the two sides of dihydropyridines is to regard the preferred conformation of the 1,4-dihydropyridine ring as a boat, with the C4 as the bow, the axial ring as the bowsprit and the nitrogen as the stern (Fig. 3). The two sides of the dihydropyridine ring can then be referred to as the port (left) and starboard (right) sides [10].

Influence of the Size of the Ester Groups

A number of enantiomers (Fig. 3, item 11) with known absolute configuration demonstrate that the more active enantiomer is the one that has the more bulky ester on the port side [5] (Fig. 3). The generality of this rule could be demonstrated in a very impressive way, by discovering two mistakes in the literature [11,12], for example, the wrong published absolute configuration of the active amlodipine enantiomer.

Conformation of the Ester Group

Rotation of both ester groups at room temperature is possible (Fig. 4). Assuming a favored coplanar arrangement of the ester carbonyl with the double bond of the 1,4-dihydropyridine ring, three conformations are possible for the ester groups, *trans/trans* (Fig. 4, item 12), *cis/trans* (Fig. 4, item 13) and *cis/cis* (Fig. 4, item 14). Analysis of the results of 26 X-ray structural investigations shows that no example with *trans/trans* conformation was detected [9]. At least one ester must be in the *cis* conformation. Fused 1,4-

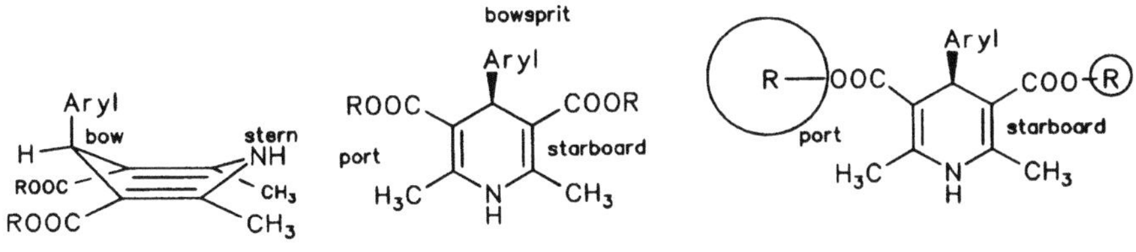

9 10 11

Fig. 3. Regarding the 1, 4-dihydropyridine as a boat and using sailing terminology, both sides of the 1,4-dihydropyridine are clearly distinguishable. In the active enantiomer the more bulky substituent is on the port

trans/trans cis/trans cis/cis

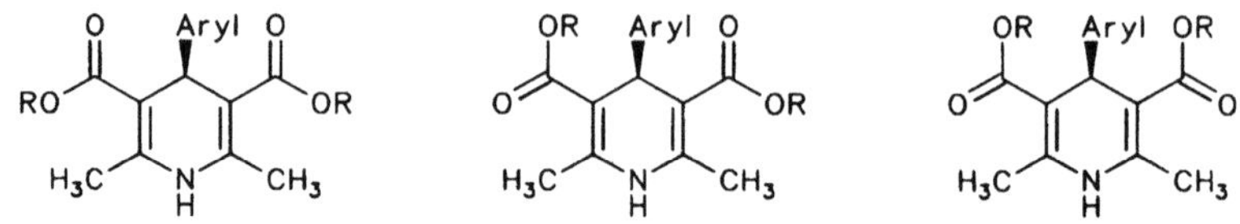

12 13 14

	12	13	14
With ortho-aryl-substituent	0	3 out of 10	7 out of 10
Without ortho-aryl-substituent	0	14 out of 16	2 out of 16

Fig. 4. Conformations of the ester groups in 1,4-dihydropyridines determined by X-ray structural analyses. (From [9])

dihydropyridines also support this hypothesis (Fig. 5). Thiophene derivatives (Fig. 5, item 15), synthesized by Shionogi, and naphthirinones (Fig. 5, item 16), synthesized by Goedecke, which can be regarded as derivatives with fixed *cis* ester conformation, exhibited potent calcium antagonistic behavior [13,14].

The pure enantiomers of structure 15 shown in Fig. 5 with known absolute configuration can answer the important questions about the nature and function of the port ester.

The *S*-enantiomer (Fig. 5, *S*-15) with the thiophene moiety on the port side is about 50 times more potent than *R*-15 (Fig. 5). The corresponding derivative with fixed "*trans* ester" conformation on the port side (Fig. 5, *S*-17) is nearly inactive ([13]; the racemate of 17 has been synthesized and showed no activity).

These examples demonstrate the importance of the *cis* conformation of the port side ester. Another important point is the ability of the ester to form hydrogen bondings to dihydropyridine receptor. The high potency of *S*-15 shows that hydrogen bonds are not essential on the port side, because the thiophene moiety is unable to form hydrogen bonds. In contrast the inactive derivatives *R*-15 and *R*-17 (Fig. 5) suggest that hydrogen bonds *are* essential on the starboard side.

To investigate the ester conformation on the starboard side, we synthesized analogues of derivative 16 [14] with known *S*-configurations (S-18 and S-19 in Fig. 5) and a "fixed ester" on the starboard side. These compounds

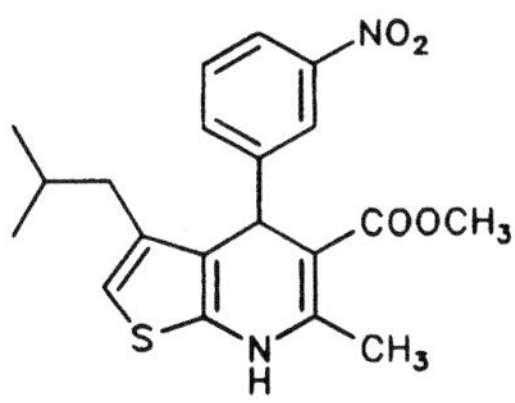

15 (active)

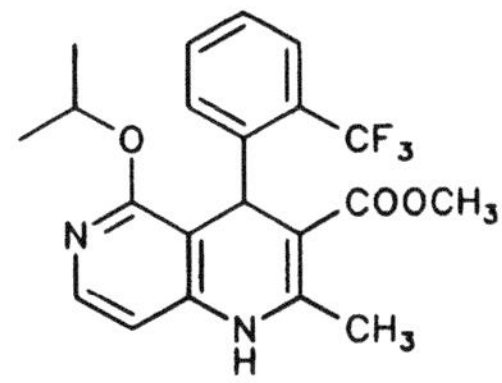

16 (active)

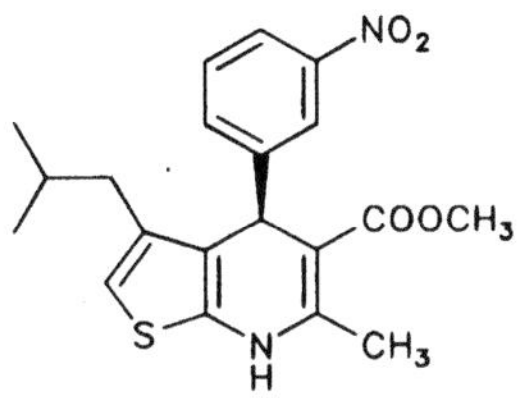

S–15 (active)

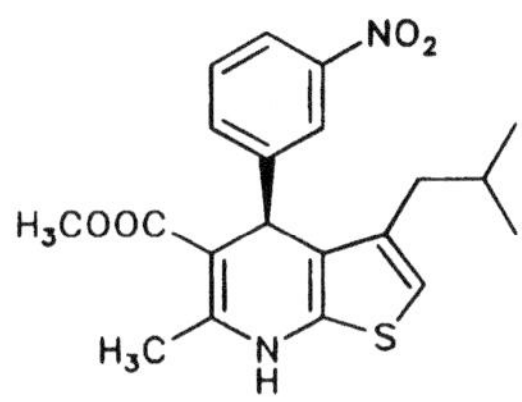

R–15 (inactive)

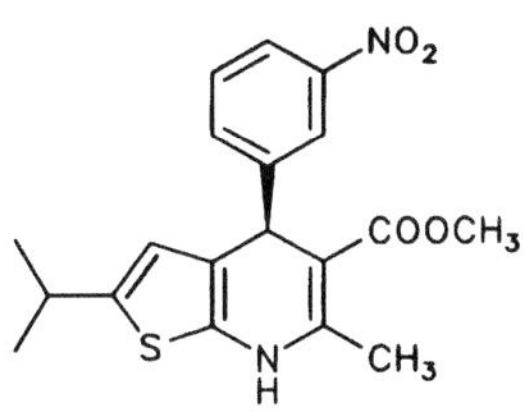

S–17 (inactive)

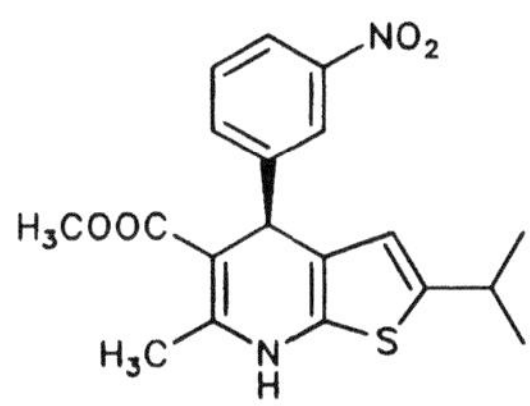

R–17 (inactive)

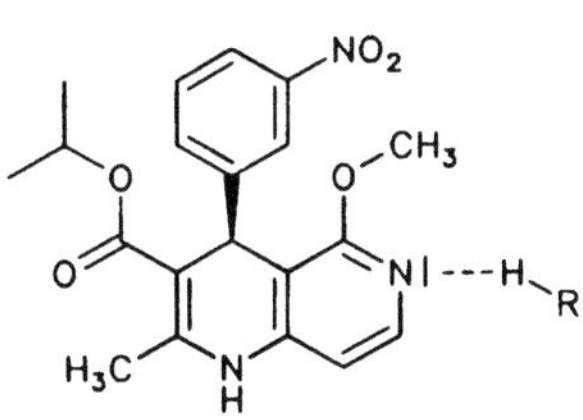

S–18 (active)

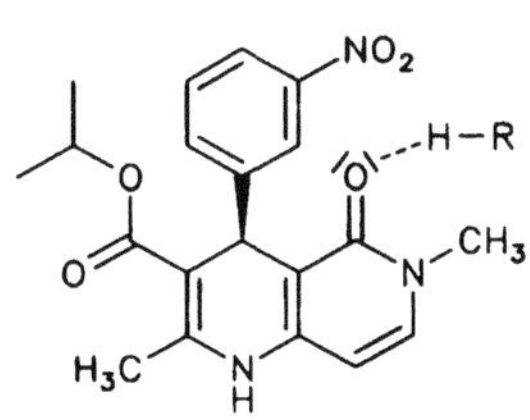

S–19 (less active)

Fig. 5. Dihydropyridines with "fixed ester" conformation

were expected to form hydrogen bonds, due to the free electron pairs of the nitrogen (in 18) or oxygen (in 19). The fixed *cis* isomer 18 is about 30 times more active than the isomer 19 shown in Fig. 5 (S. Goldmann and J. Hütter, unpublished results) and so it is likely that also the starboard ester has to be in the *cis* conformation, and – in contrast to the port side – hydrogen bonds with the dihydropyridine receptor are essential.

The facts concerning the active conformation of calcium antagonists and the likely interactions with the receptor are summarized in Fig. 7 (left side):

1. both esters are in *cis* conformation
2. both the starboard ester and the NH-proton at the bottom must form hydrogen bonds to the receptor.
3. The 4-aryl-substituent should be above the plane for optimal binding, due to a lipophilic interaction with the receptor.
4. In comparison to the starboard side, the port side is very variable, without any essential hydrogen bondings to the receptor. Bulky esters are tolerated [5] as are the amlodipine substituents in the 2-position [11].

Reversal of the Pharmacological Activity by Replacement of the Ester Function

The replacement of one ester with groups such as nitro, lactone, or hydrogen cause the agonism of the dihydropyridines. Both esters play different roles at the receptor and therefore it is very important to know which ester exchange will cause a reversal of activity. The answer can easily be given by knowledge of the absolute configuration of the active agonistic enantiomer. In Fig. 6, calcium agonistic dihydropyridines with known absolute configuration are shown: the *S*-enantiomer of BAY K 8644 (*S*-2), the Sandoz analogue *S*-20 [15], the lactone *R*-21 and the unsubstituted derivative *S*-4 ([5]; S. Goldmann and J. Hütter, unpublished results). In all these examples the port side ester must be replaced to transform antagonists into agonists. The important differences between antagonists are to be found only on the port side. The starboard side of the agonists is identical to that in the antagonists. Figure 7 shows the essential structural differences between an antagonist and an agonist. Instead of the bulky lipophilic ester on the port side, agonists have a small nitro or lactone group, inducing a negative potential in this area. The negative potential induced by the nitro group in *S*-2 (Fig. 6) or the lactone in *R*-21 (Fig. 6) is quite clear, but obviously not in the case of the unsubstituted agonist *S*-4 (Fig. 6). However, if the negative potential is the *essential* reason for agonistic activity the weak agonist *S*-4 should also exhibit a negative potential. Calculation of the potential map of derivatives of *S*-4 by Höltje et al. [16] results in a small negative potential in the same area, caused by the π-electrons of the aromatic ring [5].

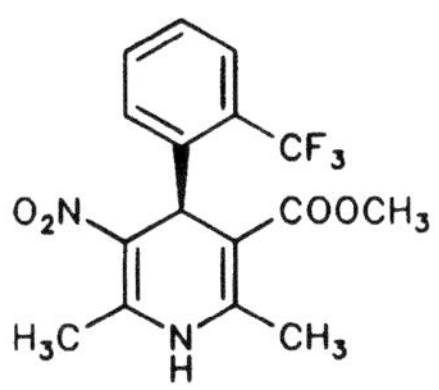

(−) S−2

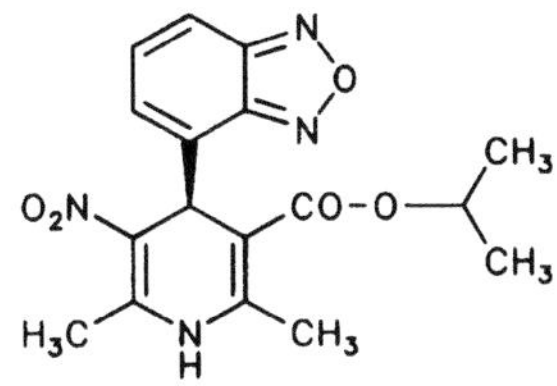

(+) S−20

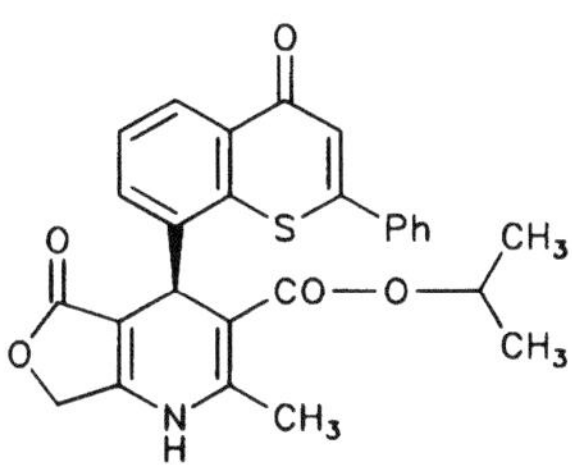

(−) R−21

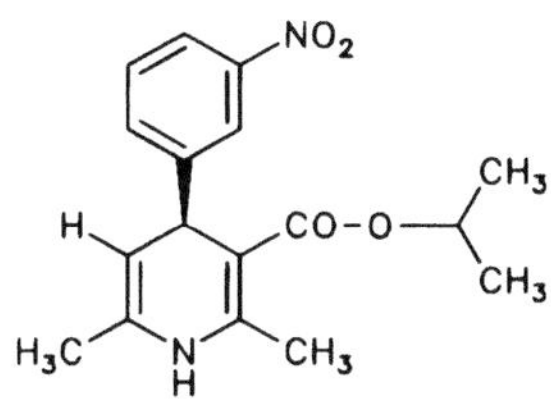

(−) S−4

Fig. 6. Calcium agonists with known absolute configuration

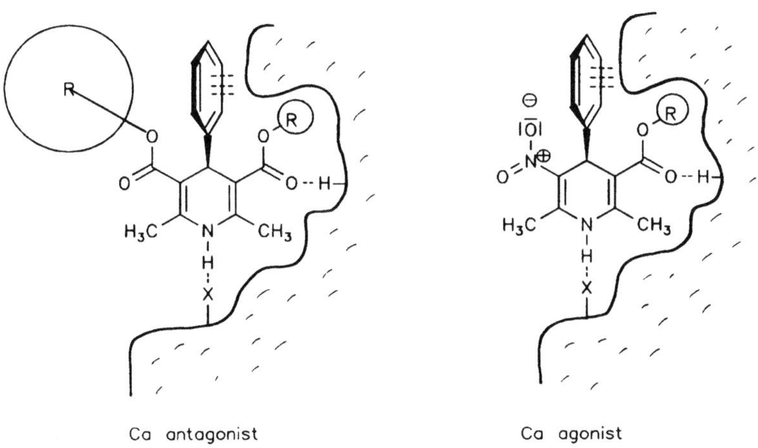

Fig. 7. Bioactive conformation and likely interactions of calcium antagonist and calcium agonist with a hypothetical receptor pocket

S-4 shows only few agonistic effects, is chemically instable and therefore not very important, but supports the importance of negative potential for agonism. For example, if the π-electrons are removed by replacing the phenyl ring with a cyclohexyl ring, the negative potential disappears and so should the agonistic effect. This is indeed the case (Fig. 8).

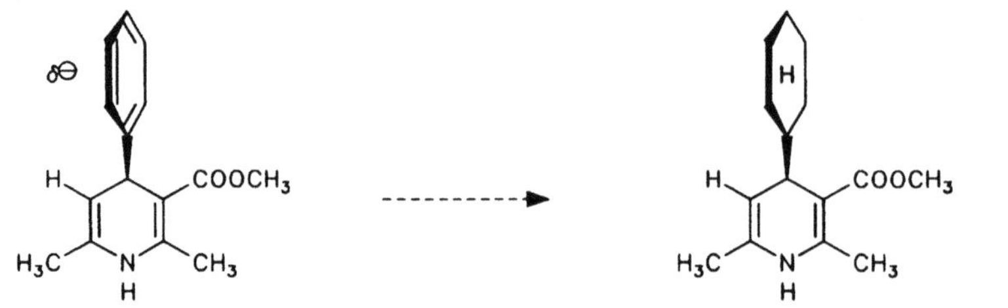

22 (weak agonist) 23 (weak antagonist)

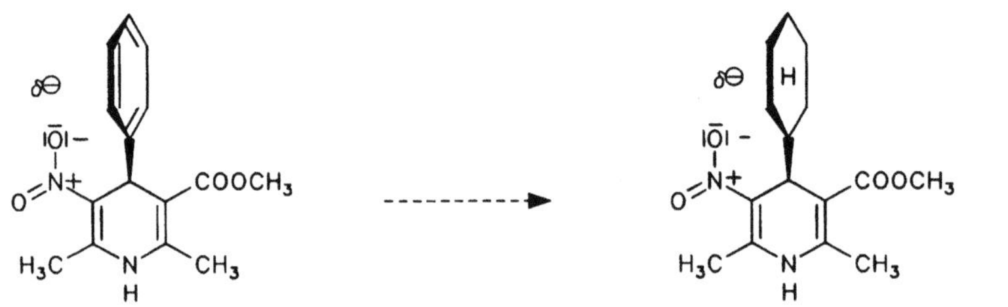

24 (agonist) 25 (agonist)

Fig. 8. Importance of the negative potential on the port side above the plane for agonism

The weak agonist 22 shown in Fig. 8 will lose the agonistic effect when the aromatic ring is changed to the cyclohexyl ring (Fig. 8-23). This is not the case when the negative potential is caused by the nitro group (Figs. 8-24, 8-25). These results indicate the importance of the negative potential in a defined area, *above* the plane on the port side of the dihydropyridine. This negative potential can be important for stabilizing positively charged parts of the receptor during opening of the calcium channel, thus stabilizing the mean open time of the channel.

Prediction of the Agonistic and Antagonistic Effects

Based on the reasons discussed above for the agonistic effects of 1,4-dihydropyridines, the surprising changes between antagonism and agonism (Fig. 1) are understandable and predictable. To induce any effect, the dihydropyridine must bind to the receptor (Fig. 7). Two hydrogen bondings – on the starboard side and at the nitrogen – are essential. In addition, lipophilic interactions with the phenyl ring above the plane are important.

A negative potential on the other side, the port side, will convert an antagonist to an agonist. *S*-2 (Fig. 1), the classical agonist, binds with the starboard ester to the receptor; the nitro group on the port side causes the negative potential and thus the agonism. *S*-4 (Fig. 1) binds and acts in similar way, but the negative potential is induced by the π -electrons of the phenyl ring above the plane. In *R*-2 and *S*-3 (Fig. 1) the nitro group plays the role of the hydrogen bond acceptor. In *R*-2 the port ester guarantees antagonism, in *S*-3 the negative potential above the plane causes weak agonism (similar to *S*-4).

In contrast, *R*-3 and *R*-4 (Fig. 1) bear no substituent on the starboard side which is able to form hydrogen bonds to the receptor. The only way to bind to the receptor is with the port side. In this case the 4-phenyl substituent is not *above* the plane and therefore no agonism will be observed.

Summary and Outlook

It is likely that, in the bioactive conformation of the calcium antagonistic dihydropyridines, both esters occupy the *cis* conformation, the more bulky ester on the port side. The smaller ester on the starboard side is important

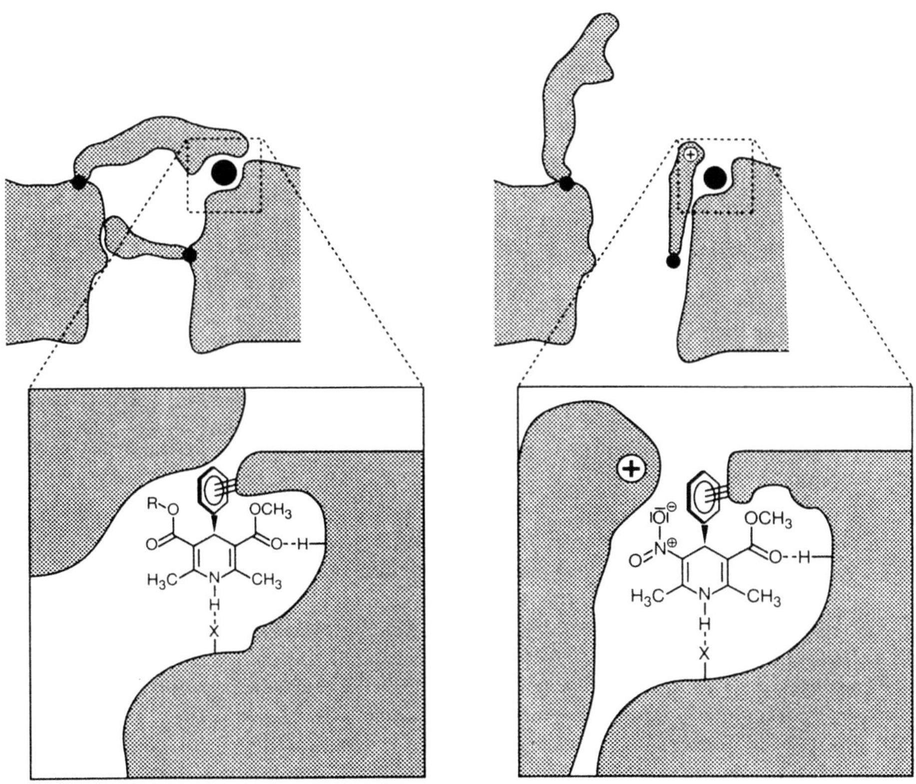

Fig. 9. *Left*, calcium antagonist stabilizes the inactive state. *Right*, calcium agonist stabilizes the open state

as a hydrogen bond acceptor. Exchange of the port ester by substituents such as nitro, hydrogen, or a 5-ring lactone will convert antagonists to agonists. It is very likely that the negative potential on the port side above the plane – induced by the nitro group, lactone, or π-electrons of the 4-aryl substituent – is essential to converting antagonists to agonists. This negative potential can be important for stabilizing positively charged parts in the open state of the calcium channel, thus prolonging the open time of the gate.

Figure 9 shows a model of the calcium channel with 1,4-dihydropyridines as modulators. The model explains in a very simplified way, the importance of the negative potential for agonists.

References

1. Schramm M, Thomas G, Towart R, Franckowiak G (1983) Novel dihydropyridines with positive inotropic action through activation of Ca^{2+}-channels. Nature 303:535
2. Franckowiak G, Bechem M, Schramm M, Thomas G (1985) The optical isomers of the 1,4-dihydropyridine Bay K 8644 show opposite effects on Ca-channels. Eur J Pharmacol 114:223–226
3. Zheng W, Stoltefuß J, Goldmann S, Triggle DJ (1992) Pharmacologic and radioligand binding studies of 1,4-dihydropyridines in rat cardiac and vascular preparations: stereoselectivity and voltage dependence of antagonist and activator interactions. Mol Pharmacol 41:535
4. Goldmann S, Stoltefuß J (1991) 1,4-Dihydropyridines: Effects of chirality and conformation on the calcium antagonist and calcium agonist activities. Ang Chem Int Ed Engl 30:1573
5. Goldmann S, Stoltefuß J (1991) 1,4-Dihydropyridines: Effects of chirality and conformation on the calcium antagonist and calcium agonist activities. Ang Chem Int Ed Engl 30:1559–1578
6. Seidel W, Meyer H, Born L, Kazda S, Dompert W (1985) Rigid calcium antagonists of the Nifedipine-type: geometric requirements for the dihydropyridine receptor. In: Seydel J (ed) QSAR and strategies in the design of bioactive compounds. Proc Eur Symp Quant Struct-Act Relat, 5th edn. VCH, Weinheim, pp 366–369
7. Baldwin JJ, Claremon DA, Lumma PK, McClure DE, Rosenthal SA, Winquist RJ, Faison EP, Kaczorowski GJ, Trumble MJ, Smith GM (1987) Diethyl 3,6-dihydro-2,4-dimethyl-2,6-methano-1,3-benzothi azocine-5,11-dicarboxylates as calcium entry antagonists: new conformationally restrained analogues of Hantzsch 1,4-dihydro pyridines related to Nitrendipine as probes for receptor-site conformation. J Med Chem 30:690–695
8. Goldmann S, Geiger W (1984) Rotational barriers of 4-aryl-1,4-dihydropyridines (Ca antagonists). Angew Chem Int Ed Engl 23:301
9. Triggle DJ, Langs DA, Janis RA (1989) Ca^{2+} channel ligands: structure-function relationships of the 1,4-dihydropyridines. Med Res Rev 9:123–180
10. Beard H, McKie R (1981) Sailing: a sailor's dictionary, Workman, New York

11. Goldmann S, Stoltefuß J, Born L (1992) Determination of the absolute configuration of the active Amlodipine enantiomer as (−)-S: a correction. J Med Chem 35:3341
12. Marciniak G, Delghado A, Leclerc G, Velly J, Decker N, Schwartz J (1989) New 1,4-dihydropyridine derivatives combining calcium antagonism and α-adrenolytic properties. J Med Chem 32:1402–1407
13. Adachi I, Yamamori T, Hiramatsu Y, Sakai K, Mihara S, Kawakami M, Masui M, Uno O, Ueda M (1988) Synthesis of 4,7-Dihydrothieno[2,3-b]-pyridines with vasodilator and antihypertensive activities. Chem Pharm Bull (Tokyo) 36:4389–4402
14. Satzinger G, Hartenstein J, Mannhardt K, Kleinschroth J, Fritschi E, Osswald H, Weinheimer G (1986) 1, 6-Naphthyridin-Derivate, Verfahren zu deren Herstellung und deren Verwendung. DE 3431 303. Goedecke AG
15. Hof RP, Rüegg UT, Hof A, Vogel A (1985) Stereoselektivity at the calcium channel: opposite action of the enantiomers of a 1,4-dihydropyridine. J Cardiovasc Pharmacol 7:689
16. Höltje HD, Marrer S (1987) A molecular graphics study on structure-action relationships of calcium-antagonistic and agonistic 1,4-dihydropyridines. J Comput-Aided Mol Des 1:23

Pharmacological Classification of High-Threshold Calcium Channels in Rat Neurons

B.P. Bean and I.M. Mintz

Introduction

Voltage-dependent calcium channels are present in all neurons. They are closed at normal resting potentials, and they open when a membrane is depolarized by an action potential. One important function of calcium channels in neurons is to mediate release of neurotransmitter from presynaptic nerve terminals. In addition, calcium channels help initiate electrical action potentials in various cell bodies and dendrites. It is very likely that calcium entry through voltage-dependent calcium channels is also important for a whole range of phenomena triggered by increases in internal calcium levels. Among these phenomena may be cell death resulting from prolonged calcium entry subsequent to long-lasting depolarizations, as may occur during ischemia.

It the last decade or so, it has become clear that mammalian neurons possess a number of different types of calcium channels, each with distinctive physiological and pharmacological properties [2–11]. Some calcium channels in mammalian brains are sensitive to classical calcium channel blockers like nitrendipine and nifedipine. However, such channels apparently make up only a small (but perhaps highly significant) fraction of total voltage-dependent calcium channels in neurons. There are few synthetic molecules that have yet been found to be effective blockers of the other types of calcium channels in neurons. Development of such molecules may be an effective route to new neuroprotective drugs.

So far, four types of calcium channels in neurons can be distinguished fairly clearly by their different physiological and pharmacological properties. We have focussed particularly on using pharmacological tools to distinguish different types of calcium channels. This article describes work we have done to distinguish different types of calcium channels in the central neurons of rat brains.

Department of Neurobiology, Harvard Medical School, 200 Longwood Avenue Boston, MA 02115, USA

T-Type Calcium Channels

T-type calcium channels (also called low voltage-activated, LVA, or low-threshold calcium channels) are characterized by their activation at relatively negative membrane potentials and by rapid inactivation kinetics [2,3]. T-type calcium channels can be easily recognized by their distinctive voltage-dependence and kinetics. They are present in many types of neurons, but often in only a small fraction of individual cells. Their pharmacology is relatively undeveloped. A variety of drug molecules have been described to block T-type channels, but all are drugs that were previously known to block other calcium channels and noncalcium channels. There is not yet a high-affinity, specific blocker of T-type calcium channels.

L-Type Calcium Channels

L-type calcium channels can be defined by their sensitivity to dihdyropyridine drugs such as nimodipine [2,3]. L-type calcium channels form most or all of the voltage-dependent calcium current in cardiac muscle and vascular

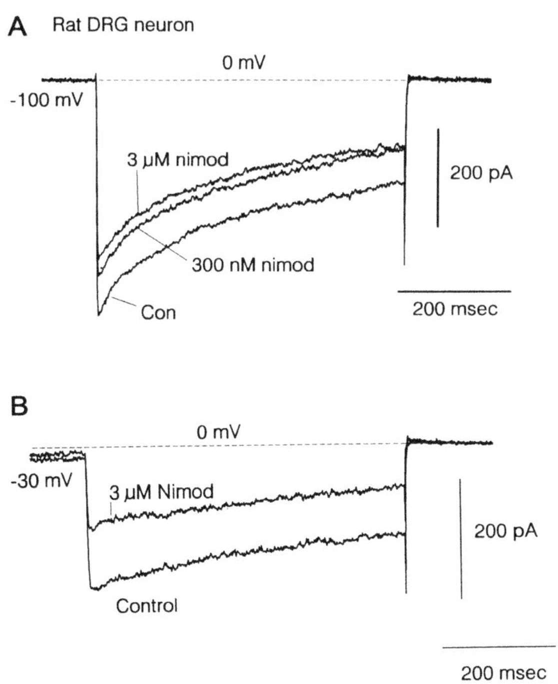

Fig. 1A,B. Nimodipine (*nimod*) inhibition of calcium channel current in a rat dorsal root ganglion neuron

muscle. Most if not all existing calcium channel blockers, including dihydropyridines, phenylalkylamines, and benzothiazepines, are targeted mainly against L-type channels. But in most neurons, L-type channels make up only a small or moderate fraction of the overall calcium current. Figure 1 shows the effects of applying two different concentrations of nimodipine to a rat dorsal root ganglion neuron while recording voltage-depdendent calcium currents. Nimodipine (300 n*M*) inhibited only about 20% of the calcium channel current elicited by depolarizing the cell membrane from −100 mV to 0 mV. Increasing the nimodipine concentration (3 μM) had only a small additional effect. The results in Fig. 1 are consistent with the presence in this neuron of a fraction of L-type current that is effectively blocked by nimodipine but that makes up only about 20%–25% of the overall calcium current elicited from a holding potential of −100 mV.

In cardiac muscle and vascular muscle, the potency with which L-type calcium channels are blocked by dihydropyridine drugs is dramatically enhanced at somewhat depolarized holding potentials. This can be interpreted as reflecting especially tight binding of drugs to the inactivated state of the calcium channel [1]. In principle, the effectiveness of nimodipine in blocking calcium channels in neurons might be greatly enhanced at depolarized holding potentials. In Fig. 1B, the effect of 3 μM nimodipine is shown when the cell is held at −30 mV rather than −100 mV. Nimodipine blocks about the same amount of absolute current elicited from the two holding potentials, although the fractional block of current elicited from −30 mV is greater because the control current is smaller than that elicited from −100 mV, A simple interpretation is that the L-type calcium channels contribute about the same amount of current from the two holding potentials (and that 3 μM nimodipine blocks this current at both holding potentials) but that other, nondihydropyridine-sensitive channels contribute substantial current from −100 mV but much less from −30 mV.

An important point from Fig. 1 is that while nimodipine-sensitive L-type current makes a relatively small contribution to overall calcium current elicited from negative holding potentials, if a neuron is steadily depolarized L-type channels may form a much greater fraction of the current (about half in the neuron of Fig. 1). McCarthy and Tanpiengco [5] have shown that nanomolar concentrations of nimodipine are capable of inhibiting L-type calcium channels in depolarized neurons. Since neurons are often depolarized under pathological conditions such as ischemia, L-type channels may be particularly important for calcium entry under such conditions. Blocking L-type channels by nimodipine may then have relatively little effect under normal conditions but be effective in reducing calcium entry in pathologically depolarized neurons. The combination of little effect on normal function and enhanced effect in pathological conditions is ideal for a therapeutically useful drug.

There is still only limited information on the detailed pharmacology of L-type calcium channels in neurons. For example, interactions of phenylalkylamines and benzothiazepines with neuronal L-type calcium channels have not been described in much detail. Since the kinetic and voltage-dependent properties of neuronal L-type calcium channels differ somewhat from those in cardiac muscle and smooth muscle, where there has been extensive work, the pharmacology of neuronal L-type channels could also be somewhat different. For example, neuronal L-type calcium channels generally show less inactivation than do calcium channels in cardiac muscle, and the properties of the inactivated state could be especially important for drug block.

N-Type Calcium Channels

N-type calcium channels were originally distinguished from L-type channels by somewhat different characteristics of voltage-dependence, kinetics, and single channel behavior [2,3]; also, N-type channels were found to be resistant to dihydropyridines.

A very effective blocker of N-type channels has been found: a peptide toxin isolated from the venom of a sea snail, *Conus geographus*. This toxin, called ω-conotoxin (ω-CgTx), blocks current through N-type calcium channels with a half-blocking concentration of approximately 30 n*M* [10]. The sensitivity of N-type calcium channels to ω-CgTx can be used to isolate the fraction of overall calcium current carried through N-type channels. The toxin is very potent in blocking N-type calcium channels but has no effect on other types of calcium channels (including L-type, P-type, and T-type channels).

Almost all of the current (typically, ~90%) in sympathetic neurons of the rat superior cervical ganglion is blocked by ω-CgTx [7,10]. However, N-type current makes up a much smaller fraction of the high-threshold current in most central neurons. In Purkinje neurons, N-type calcium current accounts for only about 5% of the current. In many other neurons, N-type current makes up 40%–50% of the high-threshold current [7,10]. Figure 2 shows a typical example of ω-CgTx applied to a central neuron. In this pyramidal neuron from the visual cortex, a saturating concentration of ω-CgTx blocked about 20% of the overall high-threshold calcium channel current.

P-Type Calcium Channels

There are other types of calcium channels in neurons besides L-type and N-type channels. This can be seen in experiments in which high concentrations of dihydropyridines and ω-CgTx are applied simultaneously. A typical example is shown in Fig. 2. In this large neuron from the visual cortex (most likely a pyramidal neuron), a large concentration (3 μ*M*) of ω-CgTx inhibited 17% of the control current; 2 μ*M* nimodipine, in the continuing

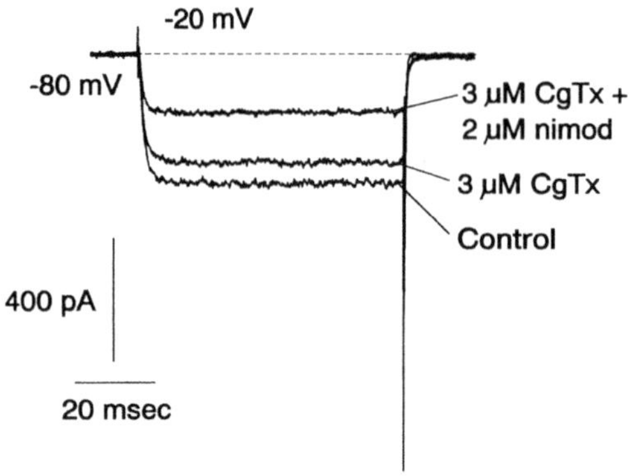

Fig. 2. Incomplete block by cumulative addition of ω-conotoxin (*CgTx*) and nimodipine (*nimod*) to a rat visual cortical neuron

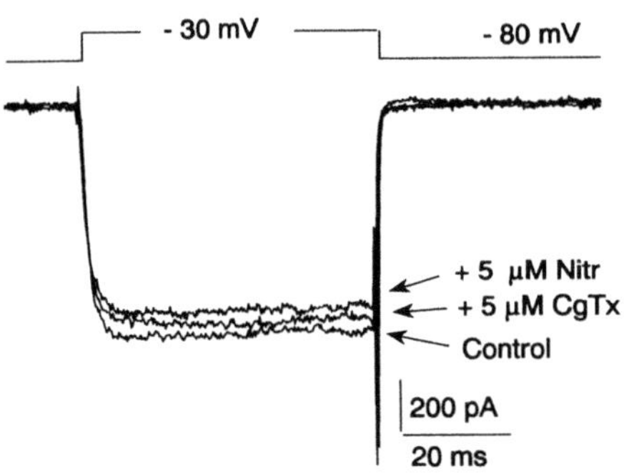

Fig. 3. Minimal effects of ω-conotoxin (*CgTx*) and nitrendipine (*Nitr*) on high-threshold calcium channel current in a rat cerebellar Purkinje neuron. (From [7])

presence of 3 μM ω-CgTx, then inhibited another 38% of the initial control current. Thus, in this central neuron L-type calcium channels contributed 38% of the calcium current, N-type channels contributed 17%, and 45% of the current flowed through channels with undefined pharmacological properties.

The calcium channel currents in Purkinje neurons are particularly interesting. Purkine neurons have low-threshold currents, carried through T-type calcium channels, and high-threshold currents [9]. Every Purkinje neuron has high-threshold current, but only a minority have T-type channels. The high-threshold current in Purkinje neurons is unusual in having very little contribution from L-type or N-type calcium channels [7–10]. A typical example is shown in Fig. 3. In this neuron, which had no T-type current, neither ω-CgTx nor nitrendipine had any significant effect on the calcium channel current, even though both were applied at high concentrations that would produce saturating block of N-type and L-type channels, respectively.

These observations support an earlier suggestion that calcium channels in cerebellar Purkinje cells are pharmacologically different from L-type and N-type channels. The name "P-type" channels was proposed for the predominant calcium channels in Purkinje neurons [4].

A substance called ω-Aga-IVA in the venom of a spider, *Agelenopsis aperta*, is a highly effective blocker of P-type channels. ω-Aga-IVA is a 48 amino acid peptide. It was identified by Dr. Michael Adams by screening different fractions of the whole venom for their ability to inhibit depolarization-induced calcium entry into rat brain synaptosomes, which, like the high-threshold calcium channel current in Purkinje neurons, is very little affected by blockers of L-type or N-type channels. After identifying blocking activity in a peptide fraction of the whole venom, a single peptide, ω-Aga-

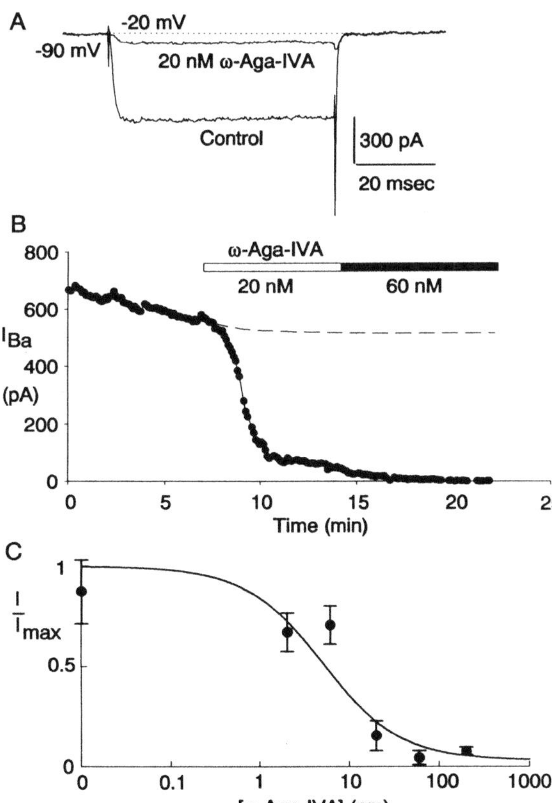

Fig. 4A–C. ω-Aga-IVA block of high-threshold calcium channel current in Purkinje neurons. (From [8])

IVA, was purified, sequenced, and characterized [8]. We found ω-Aga-IVA to be a potent and highly selective blocker of the P-type calcium channels in cerebellar Purkinje neurons. As shown in Fig. 4, only 20 n*M* ω-Aga-IVA blocks about 90% of the high-threshold current in a cerebellar Purkinje neuron. In other experiments, we found that the small fraction of current remaining in ω-Aga-IVA, usually about 10%, can be wiped out by the combination of ω-CgTx and nimodipine [7]. Dose-response experiments have shown that the half-blocking concentration of ω-Aga-IVA is about 2 n*M*.

Further experiments have shown that ω-Aga-IVA is a highly selective blocker. As shown in Fig. 5, even at concentrations as high as 100 n*M*, ω-Aga-IVA has no effect on T-type calcium channels, L-type calcium channels in either cardiac muscle cells or in neurons, or N-type calcium channels.

Based on sensitivity to ω-Aga-IVA, many other types of neurons besides Purkinje neurons appear to possess P-type calcium channels [7]. Two

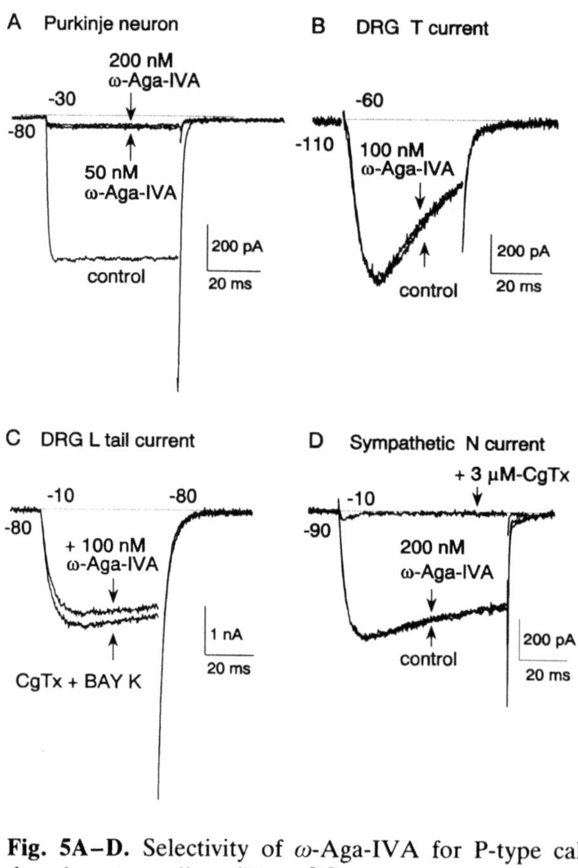

Fig. 5A–D. Selectivity of ω-Aga-IVA for P-type calcium channel current; *DRG*, dorsal root ganglion. (From [7])

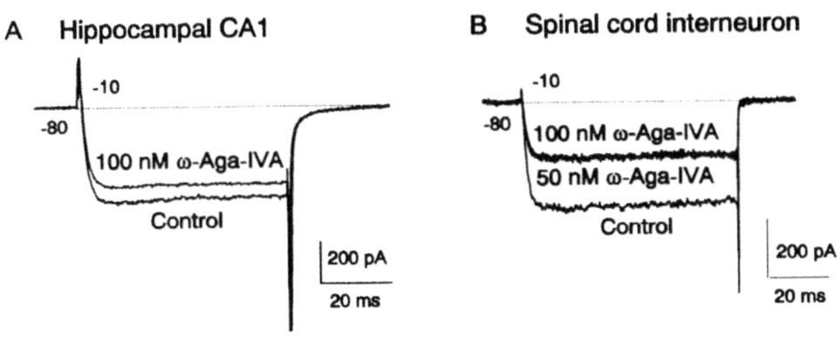

Fig. 6A,B. ω-Aga-IVA-sensitive current in a hippocampal neuron (**A**) and a spinal cord interneuron (**B**). (From [7])

Table 1. High-threshold calcium channel types in rat neurons, given as percent of current per type of cell

	P type	N type	L type	Remaining
Purkinje	92 ± 2	5 ± 1	5 ± 2	0
Hippocampal CA1	26 ± 4	37 ± 3	19 ± 3	Present
Hippocampal CA3	14 ± 4	21 ± 2	36 ± 6	25 ± 6
Visual cortex	32 ± 4	32 ± 7	23 ± 6	Present
Spinal cord	45 ± 6	34 ± 3	18 ± 5	Present
DRG	23 ± 4	43 ± 3	18 ± 2	18 ± 4
Sympathetic	0	93 ± 4	7 ± 4	0

DRG, dorsal root ganglion.

examples are shown in Fig. 6. In a hippocampal neuron, ω-Aga-IVA blocked about 20% of the high-threshold current, and in a spinal cord interneuron, ω-Aga-IvA blocked about 50% of the current.

Almost all types of central neurons possess some fraction of current sensitive to ω-Aga-IVA (Table 1). In hippocampal CA1 neurons, spinal cord interneurons, and visual cortical neurons, virtually every neuron has at least some current sensitive to ω-Aga-IVA and thus defined as P-type current. As judged by sensitivity to ω-Aga-IVA, the expression or P-type channels varies in different brain regions. About 25% of the hippocampal CA3 neurons we have tested had no P-type current (with P-type current making up an average of only 14% of the total high-threshold calcium channel current), while every spinal cord interneuron tested had substantial P-type current, which made up an average of 45% of the overall high-threshold current. It is interesting that the two cell types with the largest fractional contribution or P-type current (at least among those we have tested so far) are cerebellar Purkinje neurons (92%) and spinal cord inter-neurons (45%), both of which are GABAergic inhibitory neurons [7].

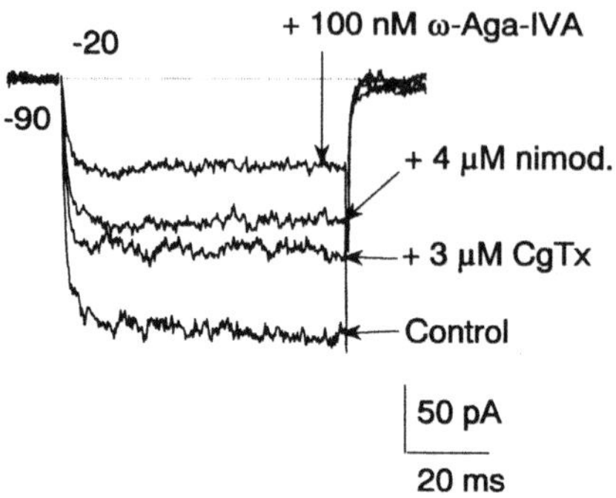

Fig. 7. Current resistant to blockers of L-type, N-type, and P-type calcium channels. Visual cortical neuron

Undefined Channel Types

In many neurons, application of saturating concentrations of nimodipine, *ω*-CgTx, and *ω*-Aga-IVA still leaves some high-threshold calcium channel current unblocked. An example is the visual cortical neurons in Fig. 7, where about 25% of current remains unblocked in the presence of all three blockers. This may represent still other channel types distinguishable from N-type, L-type, and P-type channels. Another possibility is that this current is in some sense N-type current resistant to *ω*-CgTx, L-type current resistant to nimodipine, or P-type current resistant to *ω*-Aga-IVA. Each blocker is known to be capable of producing complete block of its target current under some circumstances, but whether this is true in every neuron remains to be seen.

Synthetic Blockers

It would be of great interest to identify synthetic drug molecules that are able to inhibit N-type and P-type calcium channels. While there is a rich pharmacology of such drugs for L-type calcium channels, including the well-known drugs of the dihydropyridine, phenylalkylamine, and benzothiazepine classes, there are no potent synthetic blockers yet identified for N-type and P-type channels. Probably this is because existing calcium channel blockers were identified by screening assays using elements of the cardiovascular system, where there are no N-type or P-type channels contributing to calcium channel function. The lack of N-type and P-type channels in cardiac and vascular muscle offers appealing possibilities, because it makes it seem likely that drugs selective for N-type or P-type channels might have few side effects on cardiovascular function.

While the high-affinity block by ω-CgTx and ω-Aga-IVA allows the identification of N-type and P-type channels, these large peptides are not suitable for many kinds of experiments. Many clinically useful drugs that interact with voltage-dependent ion channels show the property of state-dependent binding. This is true of both local anesthetic block of sodium channels and dihdyropyridine block of L-type calcium channels. Such an interaction makes possible a situation in which channel block can be minimal under normal circumstances (e.g., at normal resting potentials) but can be accentuated under pathological conditions (e.g., steady depolarization). It would be particularly interesting to identify drug molecules that interact with P-type and N-type channels in such a manner. Since the gating machinery of these channels is likely to be generally similar to those of L-type channels and sodium channels, compounds that interact with the gating properties of these channels may provide a useful starting place for developing new drug molecules specific for N-type and P-type channels.

References

1. Bean BP (1984) Nitrendipine block of cardiac calcium channels: high-affinity binding to the inactivated state. Proc Natl Acad Sci USA 81:6388–6392
2. Fox AP, Nowycky MC, Tsien RW (1987) Single-channel recordings of three types of calcium channels in chick sensory neurones. J Physiol (Lond) 394:173–200
3. Fox AP, Nowycky MC, Tsien RW (1987) Single-channel recordings of three types of calcium channels in chick sensory neurones. J Physiol (Lond) 394:149–172
4. Llinas R, Sugimori M, Lin JW, Cherksey B (1989) Blocking and isolation of a calcium channel from neurons in mammals and cephalopods utilizing a toxin fraction (FTX) from funnel-web spider poison. Proc Natl Acad Sci USA 86: 1689–1693
5. McCarthy R, Tanpiengco P (1992) Multiple types of high-threshold calcium channels in rabbit sensory neurons: high-affinity block of neuronal L-type by nimodipine. J Neurosci 12:2225–2234
6. Miller RJ (1992) Voltage sensitive Ca^{2+} channels. J Biol Chem 267:1403–1406
7. Mintz IM, Adams ME, Bean BP (1992) P-type calcium channels in central and peripheral neurons. Neuron 9:1–20
8. Mintz IM, Venema VJ, Swiderek K, Lee T, Bean BP, Adams ME (1992) P-type calcium channels blocked by the spider toxin ω-Aga-IVA. Nature 355:827–829
9. Regan LJ (1991) Voltage-dependent calcium currents in Purkinje cells from rat cerebellar vermis. J Neurosci 11:2259–2269
10. Regan LJ, Sah DW, Bean BP (1991) Ca^{2+} channels in rat central and peripheral neurons: high-threshold current resistant to dihydropyridine blockers and omegaconotoxin. Neuron 6:269–280
11. Tsien RW, Ellinor PT, Horne WA (1991) Molecular diversity of voltage-dependent Ca^{2+} channels. Trends Pharmacol Sci 12:349–354

Effects of Dihydropyridine Calcium Antagonists upon Microvascular Function Following Ischemia and Oxidative Stress

J.A. Watts

Protection by Cardiodepressant Mechanisms

Many calcium antagonists are protective in experimental models of ischemia and reperfusion when used at concentrations which induce myocardial depression before the induction of ischemia (Nayler 1988). The components of protection probably involve a combination of several factors occurring during the ischemic period. These factors include energy preservation (Watts et al. 1980), decreased accumulation of cytosolic calcium and lactic acid (Watts et al. 1990a; Amende et al. 1992), reduced tissue acidosis (Ichihara and Abiko 1982), and reduced the release of catecholamines (Nayler and Sturrock 1983). The hearts receiving calcium antagonists recover greater contractile function during reperfusion than hearts receiving no drug treatment. These protected hearts have increased tissue ATP and decreased calcium overload (Watts et al. 1980; Zografos and Watts 1990), improved mitochondrial function (Watts et al. 1987a), reduced lysosomal rupture (Ichihara et al. 1987) and reduced incidence of arrhythmia (Nayler 1988) upon reperfusion. The degree of recovery of contractile function following ischemia and reperfusion is in proportion to the degree of depression of preischemic contractile function in hearts treated with verapamil (Watts et al. 1985) or diltiazem (Watts and Maiorano 1987). A comparison of equidepressant concentrations of nifedipine, verapamil, diltiazem, and buffer containing low calcium content indicates that there is no significant difference in the ability of these treatments to improve the recovery of contractile function in isolated, perfused rat hearts (Watts et al. 1986). This cardiodepressant mode of protection has been observed in many models of experimental ischemia and reperfusion if the calcium antagonists are used prophylactically (Nayler 1988).

Department of Biology, University of North Carolina at Charlotte, Charlotte, NC 28223, USA

Protection that is Independent of Cardiodepression

Dihydropyridine calcium antagonists are more selective for vascular tissue than for myocardial tissue (Ohtsuka et al. 1989). Nisoldipine shows a particularly high degree of selectivity for vascular tissue (Kazda et al. 1980; Godfraind et al. 1988; Ohtsuka et al. 1989; Deleu and Baviere 1992). Thus, using nisoldipine, it should be possible to test if a vascular selective calcium antagonist can provide protection of ischemic and reperfused hearts that is independent of cardiodepression. Experiments indicate that low (nanomolar) concentrations of nisoldipine improve the recovery of cardiac function following ischemia without decreasing preischemic contractile function or myocardial oxygen demand. These results were obtained using in vivo models of regional ischemia in cats (Mentley et al. 1988), dogs (Tumas et al. 1985; Schipke et al. 1988) and pigs (Sassen et al. 1991).

Our experiments examined the effects of pretreatment with nisoldipine (1 n*M*) upon injury from ischemia and reperfusion in isolated working rat hearts. The model was 33 min of zero flow, global ischemia, followed by 30 min of reflow. Nisoldipine treatment improved the recovery of cardiac function and tissue ATP levels. The beneficial effects of nisoldipine were not due to changes in afterload or preload (isolated perfused heart), collateral flow (zero flow model), energy preservation during ischemia (no contractile depression before ischemia, no enhancement of tissue ATP during ischemia), reduction in lactate accumulation during ischemia, or change in development of contracture during ischemia (Watts et al. 1987b, 1990b). The improved recovery of contractile function in these nisoldipine treated hearts was associated with improved reperfusion of myocardial tissue.

Effects of Nisoldipine upon no Reflow Following Ischemia

The recovery of coronary flow during reperfusion was 31% higher in nisoldipine treated hearts than in hearts that received no drug treatment (Watts et al. 1987b). The pattern of reperfusion was examined using fluorescein distribution and by measuring energy levels in subendocardial and subepicardial tissue following transient ischemia. The perfusion defect was observed in the subendocardial muscle of hearts receiving no drug treatment and averaged 15.9% ± 4.5% of the ventricular cross-sectional area. In contrast, nisoldipine treated hearts showed an area of no reflow that was significantly smaller (1.0% ± 0.9%). In addition, the subendocardial ATP and creatine phosphate levels were significantly decreased in reperfused hearts that received no drug treatment, while nisoldipine treated hearts had significantly improved levels of both high energy compounds in the subendocardial muscle layer (Watts et al. 1990b). These data indicate that nisoldipine improved the reperfusion of the subendocardial muscle layer following ischemia (fluorescein distribution) and salvaged myocardial cells

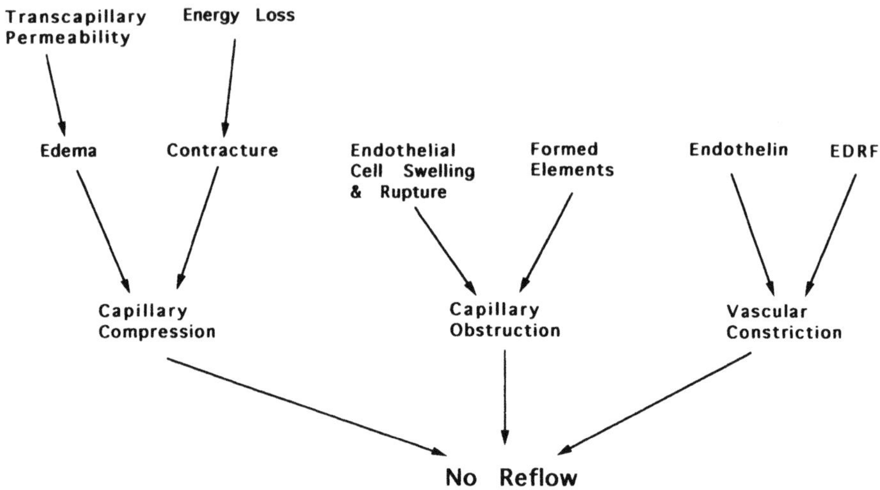

Fig. 1. Some possible causes of no reflow following transient ischemia in myocardial tissue. *EDRF*, endothelial-derived relaxing factor

in this region (increased energy levels). Additional experiments were performed to examine the processes that limit reperfusion and to understand how nisoldipine improves reflow. The failure of tissue to reperfuse after a transient ischemic period has been called the no reflow phenomenon. In cardiac tissue, the no reflow area is in the subendocardial muscle. The no reflow phenomenon may be due to capillary compression, capilllary obstruction, or changes in vascular tone (Fig. 1).

Capillary Compression

During reperfusion, capillary compression could occur by edema and myocyte swelling subsequent to increased transcapillary permeability, or by myocardial contracture resulting from decreased tissue energy levels. Transcapillary permeability to albumin increases during reperfusion of ischemic hearts (Tilton et al. 1991). Osmotically obligated water movement could cause tissue edema and compression of the capillaries. Early studies of the effects of nisoldipine upon the rise in transcapillary albumin permeability indicated that nisoldipine reduced the leak of albumin into tissue (McDonagh and Roberts 1986), however, the concentration of nisoldipine employed in that study was high (micromolar) and not clinically relevant. More recent studies indicate that the rise in coronary resistance in isolated rabbit hearts was reduced by low concentrations of nisoldipine (5 n*M*), but the rise in albumin permeability was unchanged by the drug treatment (Tilton et al. 1991). It is, therefore, unlikely that the reduction in coronary resistance observed in nisoldipine treated hearts is due to changes in tissue edema. While cardiodepressant concentrations of nisoldipine would be expected to delay the loss of high energy compounds, tissue ATP and creatine phosphate levels were not preserved during ischemia by low levels of nisoldipine (1 n*M*) (Watts et al. 1987b, 1990b). The development of ischemic contracture was not delayed by this low concentration of nisoldipine, although high concentrations of nisoldipine (300 n*M*) clearly delayed the development of contracture. Therefore, it is unlikely that the reduction in coronary resistance in nisoldipine treated hearts is due to changes in capillary compression from either myocardial contracture or edema.

Capillary Obstruction

Physical blockage of coronary arteries could occur by plugging the arteries with formed elements or by endothelial cell swelling or rupture. The contribution of the formed elements to the development of areas of no reflow should not be minimized (Lucchesi et al. 1987). The isolated hearts that were perfused with Krebs buffer showed the development of areas of no reflow without the presence of blood cells, indicating that these cells were not necessary for the formation of no reflow. Electron microscopic examination of coronary endothelial cells following 30–33 min of ischemia indicates occasional areas of endothelial cell swelling, but this is not a consistent pattern of injury in the hearts (J.A. Watts, unpublished observation). Longer (45 min) periods of ischemia followed by reperfusion caused endothelial cell swelling, bleb formation, and blockage of capillary flow (Maxwell and Gavin 1992). The effects of dihydropyridine calcium antagonists upon endothelial cell swelling after ischemia have not been examined. We have examined the rupture of endothelial cells by quantifying the release of the marker enzyme xanthine oxidase/dehydrogenase (Hawes and Watts 1992). The results indicate that the release of this enzyme activity was not significantly increased following 30 min of zero flow global ischemia and was only slightly increased following 45 min of ischemia in isolated rat hearts. The maximum release of xanthine oxidase/dehydrogenase in ischemic and reperfused hearts was small compared to the release induced by digitonin perfusion (26-fold increase in an equivalent volume of effluent) and was nearly 1000-fold less than the enzyme activity measured in tissue homogenates (Hawes and Watts 1992). Endothelial cell damage determined by enzyme release is negligible during times of ischemia that cause severe damage to myocardial contractility. While structural changes in endothelial cells may be minimal following our model of ischemia and reperfusion, functional changes in endothelial cells are profound.

Vascular Tone

The balance between signals for constriction and dilation could be altered during reperfusion. If there is a shift toward the constrictor side of this balance, either by enhanced constrictor release or response, or by inhibition of dilation responses, the coronary resistance would increase during reperfusion. This change in balance could account for the development of no reflow. Our experiments have examined the changes in constrictor responses to endothelin and dilator responses to endothelium-derived relaxing factor (EDRF) following ischemia and reperfusion in isolated rat hearts.

Endothelin

Endothelin-1 is a potent and long-lasting vasoconstrictor peptide (Yanagasawa et al. 1988). Recent experiments indicate that levels of endothelin-1 increase in human myocardial infarction (Miyauchi et al. 1991) and in several experimental models of pathology (Hieda and Gomez-Sanchez 1990; Marguiles et al. 1990; Tsuji et al. 1991; Douglas et al. 1991; Nakamura et al. 1991; Stewart et al. 1991; Matsuyama et al. 1991). An exciting observation is that antibodies to endothelin-1 reduced the size of myocardial infarcts in rats (Watanabe et al. 1991). Therefore, endothelin is released following ischemia and reperfusion and can modulate the development of injury.

We have found that the vasoconstrictor responses to endothelin-1 are significantly increased following ischemia (30 min) and reperfusion (30 min) in isolated, perfused rat hearts. The rise in sensitivity to endothelin-1 was significantly attenuated in hearts that received 1 n*M* or 5 n*M* nisoldipine before ischemia, throughout ischemia, and reperfusion (Fig. 2). These

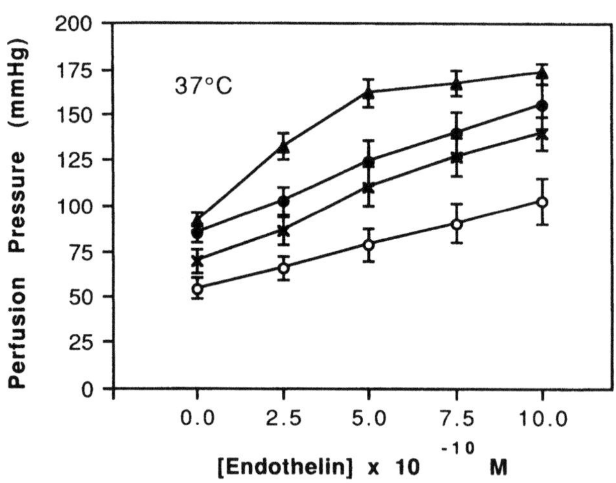

Fig. 2. Effects of endothelin-1 on perfusion pressure in control hearts treated with nisoldipine (1 n*M*, *open circles*, $n = 5$) and in hearts that were made ischemic (30 min) and reperfused with buffer containing no drug (*solid triangles*, $n = 8$), 1 n*M* nisoldipine (*solid circles*, $n = 7$), or 5 n*M* nisoldipine (*X*, $n = 7$). Values are mean ± S.E. (From Watts et al. 1992)

findings were observed when the ischemic period occurred at 37°C or at 34°C. The reduction in endothelin-1 sensitivity by nisoldipine cannot be accounted for by simple blockade of endothelin-1 responses in smooth muscle cells since control heart responses to endothelin-1 were the same in the absence or presence of nisoldipine. The rise in endothelin-1 sensitivity following ischemia and reperfusion in addition to the increased release of endothelin-1 could account for the rise in coronary resistance to flow which leads to the no reflow phenomenon. The observation that nisoldipine blunted the rise in sensitivity to endothelin-1 (Watts et al. 1992) and improved reperfusion (Watts et al. 1990b) is consistent with this hypothesis.

The mechanism of the increased sensitivity to endothelin-1 is presently under investigation. Liu et al. (1990) showed an increase in endothelin-1 receptor density (B_{max}) in membranes isolated from ischemic and reperfused rat hearts. We have not observed an increase in receptor density (B_{max}) or affinity (K_d) for endothelin-1 in membranes isolated from ischemic and reperfused rat hearts (Watts et al. 1992). This conflict of findings is, as yet, unresolved.

An alternative explanation for the increased sensitivity to endothelin-1 is that there is a decrease in endothelium-dependent dilation response following ischemia and reperfusion. Several studies indicate that endothelin-1 also triggers the release of EDRF (Topouzis et al. 1991; Takayanagi et al. 1991) via the ETb receptors present on endothelial cells (Fig. 3). The effects of endothelin-1 may normally be tempered by the release of EDRF that is triggered by endothelin-1 or by the basal release of EDRF. Dysfunction

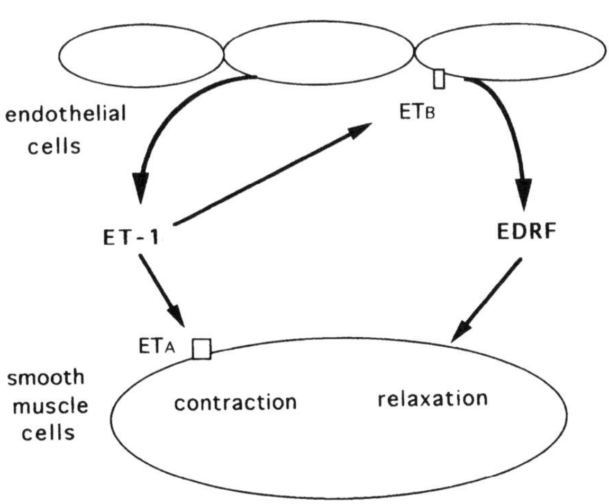

Fig. 3. Contraction induced in smooth muscle cells by the action of endothelin-1 upon ET_A receptors in the smooth muscle and the release of endothelial-derived relaxing factor (EDRF) and subsequent relaxation of smooth muscle cells by the action of endothelin-1 upon ET_B receptors

of the EDRF response following ischemia and reperfusion would favor enhanced constrictor responses to endothelin-1 and increased resistance to flow.

Endothelium-Derived Relaxing Factor

Assessment of endothelium-dependent dilation can be made by comparing the dilator responses to acetylcholine (endothelium-dependent) with those of nitroglycerin (endothelium-independent). Experiments show that endothelium-dependent dilator responses are reduced following ischemia and reperfusion in rat hearts (Tsao and Lefer 1990; Watts et al. 1992; Yaghi and Watts 1993), dog hearts (VanBenthuysen et al. 1987; Quillen et al. 1990), pig hearts (Headrick et al. 1990) and cat hearts (Tsao et al. 1990; Ma et al. 1991). The endothelial dysfunction is caused by free radicals (Tsao and Lefer 1990).

The endothelial cell dysfunction in cardiac ischemia and reperfusion in dogs was reduced by the presence of verapamil in vivo (VanBenthuysen et al. 1987) and the dihydropyridine calcium antagonist, benidipine reduced endothelial cell damage in splanchnic ischemia in rats (Karasawa et al. 1991). We have recently examined the changes in endothelium-dependent responses in low flow ischemia and reperfusion in isolated rat hearts. Rat hearts that were subjected to ischemia (20% control flow, 30 min), followed by reperfusion (30 min), exhibited reduced dilator responses to acetylcholine (34% of preischemic response) with no significant change in dilator responses to nitroglycerin (104% of preischemic response). These results indicate that endothelium-dependent dilator responses were damaged by ischemia and reperfusion. When nisoldipine (5 n*M*) was given before ischemia, throughout ischemia and the first 5 min of reperfusion, improved responses to acetylcholine were observed (no drug, 34% of preischemic; nisoldipine, 88% of preischemic) (Fig. 4).

Therefore, the hearts that are treated with nisoldipine show reduced constriction to endothelin-1 and improved dilator responses to acetylcholine following reperfusion. The improved balance of tone toward dilation could account for the improved reperfusion observed in nisoldipine treated hearts.

Antioxidant Mechanisms

Endothelial cells may not contain voltage operated calcium channels (Mugge et al. 1991; Bossu et al. 1992), suggesting an alternate mode of protection. The preservation of endothelium-dependent responses by nisoldipine may occur by the antioxidant properties of this dihydropyridine calcium antagonist. Our recent studies indicate that treatment of isolated rat hearts with tert-butylhydroperoxide (tBHP) causes endothelium-dependent injury which is similar to that observed in ischemic and reperfused hearts since

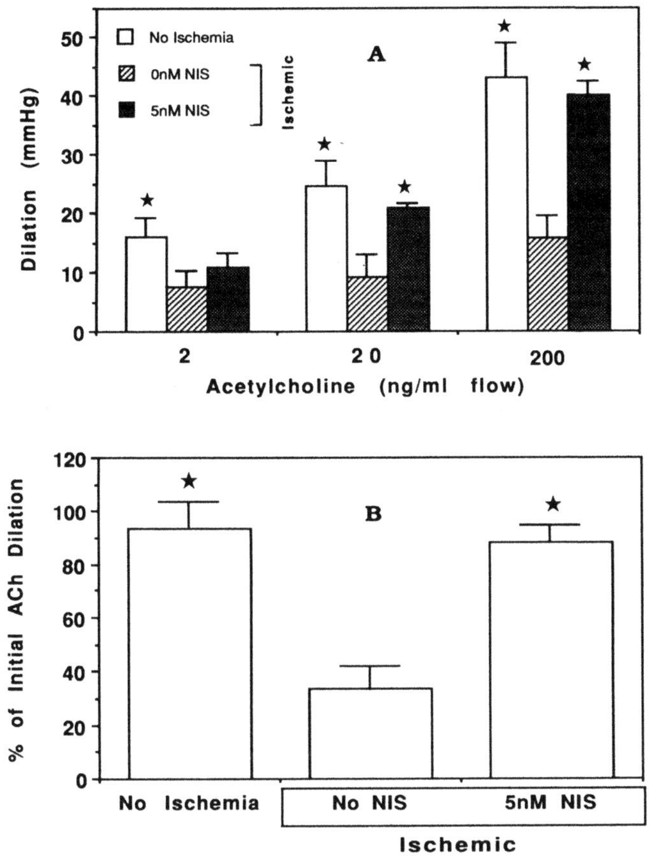

Fig. 4A,B. The coronary vessels were preconstricted with U46619 and vasodilation responses to acetylcholine were observed at the end of perfusion (**A**). Hearts received no ischemia (*clear bars*), or were made ischemic and reperfused with no drug (*hatched bars*) or 5 n*M* nisoldipine (*NIS*, *stippled bars*). Maximum responses to acetylcholine (*Ach*) at the end of perfusion are expressed as a percent of the initial response (**B**). Values are mean ± S.E., *n* = 6–8. Values with *stars* are significantly greater than values with *no stars*

responses to acetylcholine were significantly reduced (47% of pre-tBHP) while responses to nitroglycerin were unchanged. The addition of nisoldipine for 10 min before tBHP, throughout the tBHP treatment, and the first 5 min of wash improved the responses to acetylcholine in a dose-dependent manner (Fig. 5). These results indicate that nisoldipine has antioxidant activity and protects against endothelial cell dysfunction at clinically relevant concentrations.

Nisoldipine (50 n*M*) also reduced the injury to the myocardial muscle that occurred with tBHP (Nayler and Britnell 1991) and decreased the

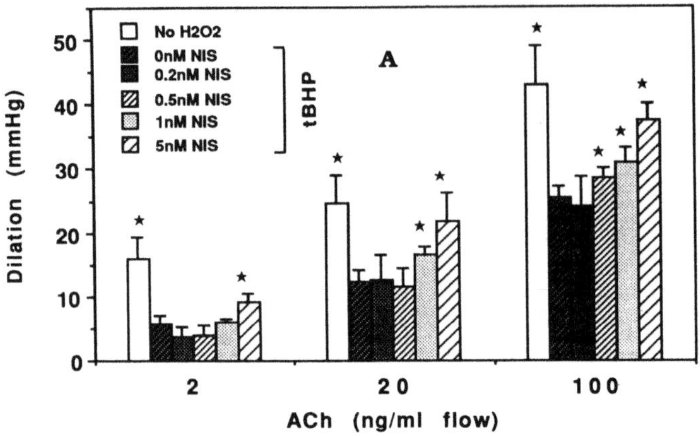

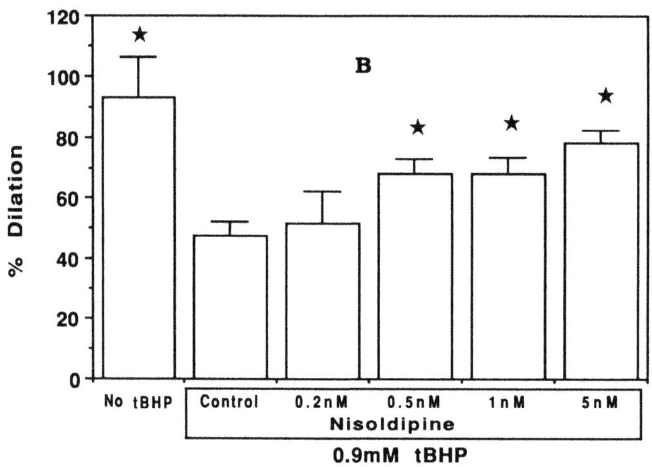

Fig. 5A,B. The coronary vessels were preconstricted with U46619 and vasodilation responses to acetylcholine were observed at the end of perfusion (**A**). Hearts received no tert-butylhydroperoxide (*tBHP*, *clear bars*), or received tBHP in the presence of the indicated concentration of nisoldipine (*NIS*). Maximum responses to acetylcholine (*Ach*) are expressed as a percent of initial responses (**B**). Values are mean ± S.E., $n = 6–8$. Values with *stars* are significantly greater than values with *no stars*

incidence of arrhythmias due to artificially generated free radicals (Li et al. 1989). Other studies have examined the antioxidant properties of calcium antagonists, but have employed high (micromolar) concentrations of these agents (Shridi and Robak 1988; Janero and Burghardt 1989; Mak et al. 1992). The dihydropyridine calcium antagonists partition most strongly into biological membranes and have the most potent antioxidant activity (Mak et al. 1992; Herbette et al. 1989). Nisoldipine has a particularly high partition into biological membranes (Janis et al. 1987; Janis and Triggle 1991) and may be expected to exert antioxidant effects at much lower concentrations. In addition to lipid partitioning, the groups attached at C-3 and C-5 of the dihydropyridine ring may be important since nisoldipine and nimodipine have similar membrane partition coefficients but nisoldipine has stronger antioxidant activity (Janero and Burghardt 1989). The concentrations of nisoldipine required to observe the antioxidant protection (0.5–5 n*M*) in our studies are the same as those required to protect against ischemia and reperfusion injury to the endothelial cells (5 n*M*) and to reduce the no reflow phenomenon (1 n*M*, Watts et al. 1990b). This concentration is also clinically relevant. Therapeutic doses of nisoldipine also reduced the peroxidation of membrane lipids in an in vivo model of ischemia in pigs (Herbaczynska Cedro and Gordon-Majszak 1990). Our additional studies show that verapamil and diltiazem do not provide antioxidant protection to endothelial cell function at 5 n*M* or 5 μM concentrations (Yaghi and Watts 1993), suggesting that these calcium antagonists are less effective in this regard.

Nisoldipine is only effective in reducing ischemic injury when it is used prophylactically. Addition of nisoldipine at the beginning of the reperfusion phase is ineffective (Watts et al. 1990b). The binding of nisoldipine to the inactivated state of calcium channels is much greater than to the resting state of the channels (Sanguinetti and Kass 1984). Perhaps nisoldipine needs to be present during ischemia when the cells would be depolarized in order to maximally bind to the channels. An alternative explanation is that the addition of nisoldipine before the induction of ischemia gives time for nisoldipine to insert into the lipid portion of the bilayer, allowing the antioxidant activity to occur during reperfusion. Adding nisoldipine only during reperfusion would not allow enough time for the nisoldipine to insert into the lipid portion of the membrane before the generation of free radicals during the early phase of reperfusion.

Summary

Low concentrations of nisoldipine (nanomolar) enhance the recovery of contractile function following transient ischemia in isolated rat hearts. The beneficial effects do not accrue from cardiodepressant mechanisms, but are associated with improved reperfusion of subendocardial muscle and salvage of myocardial tissue. These concentrations of nisoldipine have antioxidant activity that may account for the preservation of endothelium-dependent dilation and the reduction in constrictor responses to endothelin-1 after ischemia. The improvement in the balance of vascular tone toward dilation could explain how nisoldipine improves myocardial perfusion following transient ischemia. These mechanisms occur at clinically relevant concentrations of nisoldipine.

References

Amende I, Bentivegna LA, Zeind AJ, Wenzlaff P, Grossman W, Morgan JP (1992) Intracellular calcium and ventricular function. Effects of nisoldipine on global ischemia in the isovolumic, coronary-perfused heart. J Clin Invest 89:2060–2065

Bossu JL, Elhamdani A, Feltz A, Tanzi F, Aunis D, Thierse D (1992) Voltage-gated Ca entry in isolated bovine capillary endothelial cells: evidence of a new type of BAY K 8644-sensitive channel. Pflugers Arch 420:200–207

Deleu D, Bavier HV (1992) Coronary-selective properties of nisoldipine. Am Heart J 123:1726

Douglas SA, James S, Hiley CR (1991) Endothelial modulation and changes in endothelin pressor activity during hypoxia in the rat isolated perfused superior mesenteric arterial bed. Br J Pharmacol 103:1441–1448

Godfraind T, Morel N, Wibo M (1988) Mechanisms of the vascular selectivity of nisoldipine. In: Lichtlen PR, Hugenholtz PG (eds) Nisoldipine 1988. Schattauer, Stuttgart, pp 25–37

Hawes EM, Watts JA (1992) Xanthine oxidase/dehydrogenase release following ischemia in isolated rat hearts. Am J Cardiovasc Pathol (in press)

Headrick JP, Angello DA, Berne RM (1990) Effects of brief coronary occlusion and reperfusion on porcine coronary artery reactivity. Circulation 82:2163–2169

Herbaczynska-Cedro K, Gordon-Majszak W (1990) Nisoldipine inhibits lipid peroxidation induced by coronary occlusion in pig myocardium. Cardiovasc Res 24:683–687

Herbette LG, Vant Erve YMH, Rhodes DG (1989) Interaction of 1,4 dihydropyridine calcium channel antagonists with biological membranes: lipid bilayer partitioning could occur before drug binding to receptors. J Mol Cell Cardiol 21:187–201

Hieda HS, Gomez-Sanchez CE (1990) Hypoxia increases endothelin release in bovine endothelial cells in culture, but epinephrine, norepinephrine, serotonin, histamine and angiotensin II do not. Life Sci 47:247–251

Ichihara K, Abiko Y (1982) Effect of diltiazem, a calcium antagonist, on myocardial pH in ischemic canine heart. J Pharmacol Exp Ther 222:720–725

Ichihara K, Haneda T, Onodera S, Abiko Y (1987) Inhibition of ischemia-induced subcellular redistribution of lysosomal enzymes in the perfused rat heart by the calcium entry blocker, diltiazem. J Pharmacol Exp Ther 242:1109–1113

Janero DR, Burghardt B (1989) Antiperoxidant effects of dihydropyridine calcium antagonists. Biochem Pharmacol 38:4344–4348

Janis RA, Triggle DJ (1991) Drugs acting on calcium channels. In: Hurwitz L, Partridge LD, Leach JK (eds) The calcium channel: its properties, function, regulation and clinical relevance. CRC Press, Boca Raton, pp 195–249

Janis RA, Shrikhande AV, Greguski R, Pan M, Scriabine A (1987) Review of nisoldipine binding studies. In: Hugenholtz PG, Meyer J (eds) Nisoldipine 1987. Springer, Berlin Heidelberg New York, pp 27–35

Karasawa A, Rochester JA, Ma XL, Lefer AM (1991) Protection of endothelial damage and systemic shock by benidipine, a calcium antagonist, in rats subjected to splanchnic ischemia and reperfusion. Circ Shock 33:135–141

Kazda S, Garthoff B, Meyer H, Schlosmann K, Stoepel K, Towart R, Vatner W, Wehinger E (1980) Pharmacology of a new calcium antagonistic compound, Isobutyl methyl 1,4-dihydro-2,6-dimethyl-4-(2-nitrophenyl)-3,5-pyridinedicarboxylate (Nisoldipine, Bay K 5552). Arzneimittelforschung 30:2144–2162

Li YL, Fu SX, Li YS (1989) Prophylactic effects of m-nisoldipine and nisoldipine on reperfusion arrhythmias exacerbated by free radical generating system in Langendorff heart of rat. Acta Pharmacol Sin 10:310–315

Liu J, Chen R, Casley DJ, Nayler WG (1990) Ischemia and reperfusion increases ^{125}I-labeled endothelin-1 binding in rat cardiac membranes. Am J Physiol 258: H829–H835

Lucchesi BR, Mickelson JK, Homeister JW, Jackson CV (1987) Interaction of the formed elements of blood with the coronary vasculature in vivo. Fed Proc 46:63–72

Ma XL, Tsao PS, Viehman GE, Lefer AM (1991) Neutrophil-mediated vasoconstriction and endothelial dysfunction in low-flow perfusion-reperfused cat coronary artery. Circ Res 69:95–106

Mak T, Boehme P, Weglicki WB (1992) Antioxidant effects of calcium channel blockers against free radical injury in endothelial cells. Circ Res 70:1099–1103

Margulies KB, Hildebrand FL, Lerman A, Perella MA, Burnett JC (1990) Increased endothelin in experimental heart failure. Circulation 82:2226–2230

Matsuyama K, Yasue H, Okumura K, Saito Y, Nakao K, Shirakami G, Imura H (1991) Increased plasma level of endothelin-1-like immunoreactivity during coronary spasm in patients with coronary spastic angina. Am J Cardiol 68:991–995

Maxwell L, Gavin J (1992) Anti-oxidant therapy improves microvascular ultrastructure and perfusion in postischemic myocardium. Microvasc Res 43:255–266

McDonagh PF, Roberts DJ (1986) Prevention of transcoronary macromolecular leakage after ischemia-reperfusion by the calcium entry blocker nisoldipine. Circ Res 58:127–136

Mentley RK, Brezinski ME, Tse E, Lefer AM (1988) Cardioprotective actions of nisoldipine in postreperfusion myocardial ischemia. Am Heart J 115:948–954

Miyauchi T, Sugishita Y, Yamaguchi I, Ajisaka R, Tomizawa T, Onizuka M, Matsuda M, Kono I, Yanagisawa M, Goto K, Suzuki N, Matsumoto H, Masaki T (1991) Plasma concentrations of endothelin-1 and endothelin-3 are altered differently in various pathophysiological conditions in humans. J Cardiovasc Pharmacol 17:S394–S397

Mugge A, Peterson T, Harrison DG (1991) Release of nitrogen oxides from cultured bovine aortic endothelial cells is not impaired by calcium channel antagonists. Circulation 83:1404–1409

Nakamura T, Kasai K, Sekiguchi Y, Banba N, Takahashi K, Emoto T, Hattori Y, Shimoda SI (1991) Elevation of plasma endothelin concentrations during endotoxin shock in dogs. Eur J Pharmacol 205:277–282

Nayler WG (1988) Calcium antagonists. Academic, New York

Nayler WG, Britnell S (1991) Calcium antagonists and tissue protection. J Cardiovasc Pharmacol 18:S1–S5

Nayler WT, Sturrock WJ (1983) An inhibitory effect of verapamil and diltiazem on the release of noradrenaline from ischemic and reperfused hearts. J Mol Cell Cardiol 16:331–344

Ohtsuka M, Yokota M, Kodama I, Yamada K, Shibata S (1989) New generation dihydropyridine calcium entry blockers: in search of greater selectivity for one tissue subtype. Gen Pharmacol 20:539–556

Quillen JE, Selke FW, Brooks LA, Harrison DG (1990) Ischemia-reperfusion impairs endothelium-dependent relaxation of coronary microvessels but does not affect large arteries. Circulation 82:586–594

Sanguinetti MC, Kass RS (1984) Voltage-dependent block of calcium channel current in calf cardiac purkinje fiber by dihydropyridine calcium channel antagonists. Circ Res 55:336–348

Sassen LMA, Bezstarosti K, Verdouw PD, Lamers JMJ (1991) Effects of nisoldipine on recovery of coronary blood flow, sarcoplasmic reticulum function and other biochemical parameters in post-ischemic porcine myocardium. Biochem Pharmacol 41:43–51

Schipke JD, Burkhoff D, Alexander J, Schaefer J, Sagawa K (1988) Effect of nisoldipine on coronary resistance, contractility and oxygen consumption of the isolated blood-perfused canine left ventricle. J Pharmacol Exp Ther 244: 1000–1004

Shridi F, Robak J (1988) The influence of calcium channel blockers on superoxide anions. Pharmacol Res Commun 20:13–21

Stewart DJ, Kubac G, Costello KB, Cernacek P (1991) Increased plasma endothelin-1 in the early hours of acute myocardial infarction. J Am Coll Cardiol 18:38–43

Takayanagi R, Kitazumi K, Takasaki C, Ohnaka K, Aimoto S, Tasaka K, Ohashi M, Nawata H (1991) Presence of non-selective type of endothelin receptor on vascular endothelium and its linkage to vasodilation. FEBS Lett 282:103–106

Tilton RG, Watts JA, Land MP, Larson KB, Sutera SP, Williamson JR (1991) Discordant effects of nisoldipine on coronary vascular resistance and permeability changes during reflow after ischemia in isolated rabbit hearts. J Mol Cell Cardiol 23:861–872

Topouzis S, Huggins JP, Pelton JT, Miller RC (1991) Modulation by endothelium of the responses induced by endothelin-1 and by some of its analogues in rat isolated aorta. Br J Pharmacol 102:545–549

Tsao PS, Lefer AM (1990) Time course and mechanism of endothelial dysfunction in isolated ischemic- and hypoxic-perfused rat hearts. Am J Physiol 259: H1660–H1666

Tsao PS, Aoki N, Lefer DJ, Johnson G, Lefer AM (1990) Time course of endothelial dysfunction and myocardial injury during myocardial ischemia and reperfusion in the cat. Circulation 82:1402–1412

Tsuji S, Sawamura A, Watanabe H, Takihara K, Park SE, Azuma J (1991) Plasma endothelin levels during myocardial ischemia and reperfusion. Life Sci 48: 1745–1749

Tumas J, Deth R, Kloner R (1985) Effects of nisoldipine, a new calcium antagonist, on myocardial infarct size and cardiac dynamics following acute myocardial infarction. J Cardiovasc Pharmacol 7:361–367

VanBenthuysen KM, McMurtry IF, Horwitz LD (1987) Reperfusion after acute coronary occlusion in dogs impairs endothelium-dependent relaxation to acetylcholine and augments contractile reactivity in vitro. J Clin Invest 79:265–274

Watanabe T, Suzuki N, Shimamoto N, Fujino M, Imada A (1991) Contribution of endogenous endothelin to the extension of myocardial infarct size in rats. Circ Res 69:370–377

Watts J, Maiorano L (1987) Effects of diltiazem upon globally ischemic rat hearts. Eur J Pharmacol 138:324–335

Watts JA, Koch CD, LaNoue KF (1980) Effects of Ca^{2+} antagonism on energy metabolism: Ca^{2+} and heart function after ischemia. Am J Physiol 238:H909–H916

Watts JA, Maiorano LJ, Maiorano PC (1985) Protection by verapamil of globally ischemic rat hearts: energy preservation, a partial explanation. J Mol Cell Cardiol 17:797–804

Watts JA, Maiorano LJ, Maiorano PC (1986) Comparison of the protective effects of verapamil, diltiazem, nifedipine, and buffer containing low calcium upon global myocardial ischemic injury. J Mol Cell Cardiol 18:255–263

Watts JA, Maiorano P, Harwell T (1987a) Comparison of the effects of bepridil and diltiazem upon globally ischemic rat hearts. Eur J Pharmacol 134:25–33

Watts JA, Whipple JP, Hatley AA (1987b) A low concentration of nisoldipine reduces ischemic heart injury: enhanced reflow and recovery of contractile function without energy preservation during ischemia. J Mol Cell Cardiol 19:809–817

Watts JA, Norris TA, London RE, Steenbergen C, Murphy E (1990a) Effects of diltiazem on lactate, ATP, and cytosolic free calcium levels in ischemic hearts. J Cardiovasc Pharmacol 15:44–49

Watts JA, Hawes EM, Jenkins SH, Williams TC (1990b) Effects of nisoldipine on the no-reflow phenomenon in globally ischemic rat hearts. J Cardiovasc Pharmacol 16:487–494

Watts JA, Chapat S, Johnson DE, Janis RA (1992) Effects of nisoldipine upon vasoconstrictor responses and binding of endothelin-1 in ischemic and reperfused rat hearts. J Cardiovasc Pharmacol 19:929–936

Yaghi MM, Watts JA (1993) Effects of nisoldipine upon endothelial dysfunction following ischemic and peroxidative injury in perfused rat hearts. Cardiovasc Res 27:990–996

Yanagisawa M, Inoue A, Ishikawa T, Kasuya Y, Kimura S, Kumagaye SI, Nakajima K, Watanabe TX, Sakakibara S, Goto K, Masaki T (1988) Primary structure, synthesis, and biological activity of rat endothelin, an endothelium-derived vasoconstrictor peptide. Proc Natl Acad Sci 85:6964–6967

Zografos P, Watts JA (1990) Shifts in calcium in ischemic and reperfused rat hearts: a cytochemical and morphometric study of the effects of diltiazem. Am J Cardiovasc Pathol 3:155–165

Calcium Agonists

R. Gross, M. Bechem, S. Hebisch, J. Hütter, P. Rounding, and
M. Schramm

Introduction

Dihydropyridines (DHPs), as exemplified by nifedipine (Vater et al. 1972), have become known as very powerful calcium antagonists and are important drugs in cardiovascular medicine. The discovery of DHPs with an agonistic action at the calcium channel opposite to that of the clinically widely used calcium antagonists has greatly enhanced our understanding how the calcium channel works (see Bechem et al. 1988). The prototype of these so-called calcium agonists, BAY K 8644 (Schramm et al. 1983), has been intensively investigated and proven to be a valuable pharmacological tool (Bechem et al. 1988). But none of the compounds reported on so far have been suitable for clinical use, mainly because they produce unacceptable vasoconstriction.

Hemodynamic Effects

Instead of decreasing systolic Ca^{2+} influx into the cell, as seen with calcium antagonists, calcium agonists increase it (Schramm et al. 1985; Hwang and van Breemen 1985); in this way they act as positive inotropics and vasoconstrictors. This can be seen in the experiment in an anesthetized dog shown in Fig. 1. Intravenous injection of 30 μg/kg BAY K 8644 increases systolic and diastolic blood pressure and leads to a marked increase of the rate of rise of left ventricular pressure ($LV(dP/dt)_{max}$), which can be viewed as an index of left ventricular inotropy. After a transient fall in coronary blood flow, in the face of increasing arterial blood pressure there is an increase in coronary blood flow which is probably metabolically mediated. All the hemodynamic effects of BAY K 8644 in this experiment could readily be antagonized by injection of the same dose of nifedipine.

A dose-response curve for BAY K 8644 in conscious, chronically instrumented dogs is shown in Fig. 2. There is a dose-dependent increase of

Institut für Herz-Kreislauf- und Arterioskleroseforschung, Bayer AG, Postfach 10 17 09, 42096 Wuppertal, Germany

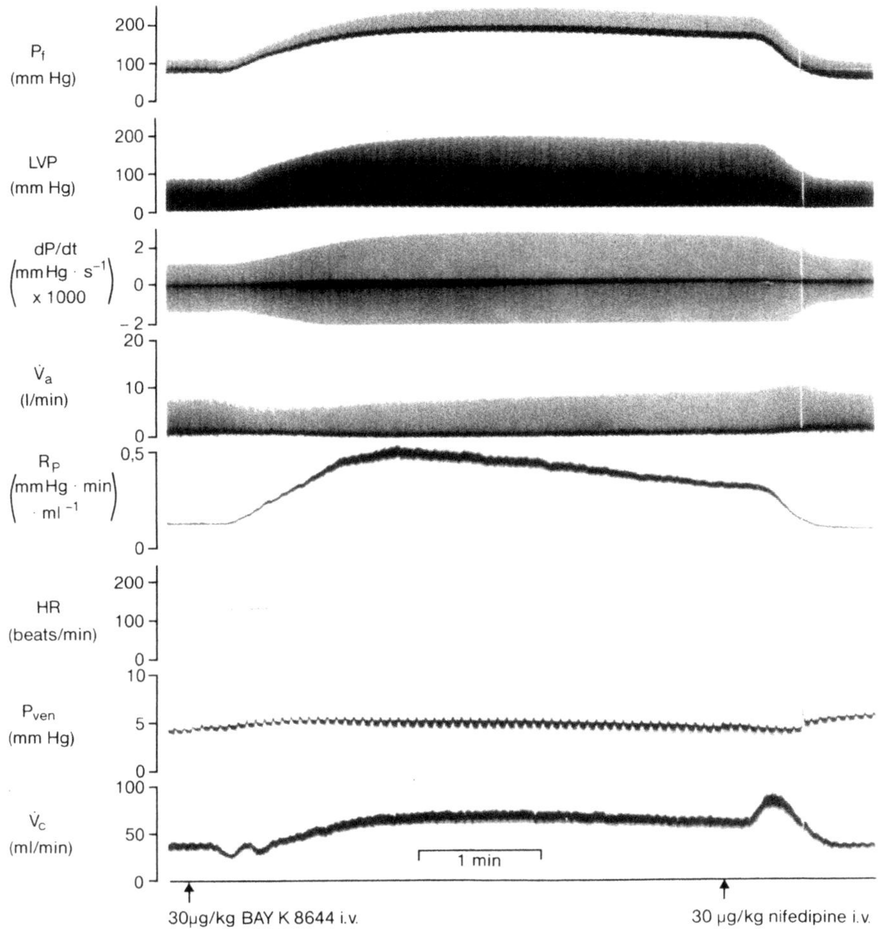

Fig. 1. Effect of an intravenous injection of 30 μg/kg BAY K 8644 into an anesthetized dog on hemodynamics (P_f, pressure in the femoral artery; *LVP*, left ventricular pressure; *dP/dt*, left ventricular rate of pressure rise; R_P peripheral resistance; *HR*, heart rate; P_{ven}, Central venous pressure; V_c, mean coronary blood flow) and its reversal by intravenous injection of 30 μg/kg nifedipine. (From Gross et al. 1985a)

$LV(dP/dt)_{max}$ from 4 μg/kg, which despite the pressoreceptor reflex-mediated bradycardia reached about 5600 mm Hg/s. Arterial blood pressure markedly increased to 196/138 mm Hg and heart rate dropped to 52/min at the highest dose given. Essentially the same dose-reponse relationship was obtained when the heart rate was kept constant at 150/min by ventricular pacing (Gross et al. 1985b). The marked increase of total peripheral resistance and the concomitant pressure increase underline the need for cardioselective calcium agonists if these compounds, apart from being valuable tools for basic research, are to be of value in the clinic.

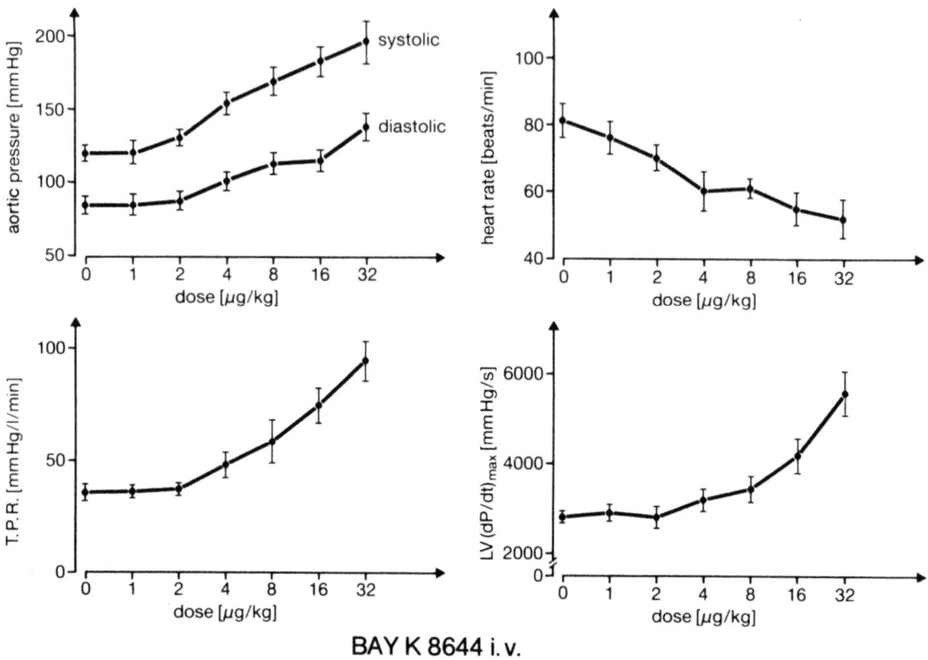

Fig. 2. Sinus rhythm. Dose-response curves for the hemodynamic effects of intravenous BAY K 8644 in seven conscious dogs. The means with their standard errors are given. (From Gross et al. 1985b)

After the enantiomers of BAY K 8644 had been separated, it became evident that the calcium agonistic principle resides in the (−)-enantiomer, while the (+)-enantiomer acts about 30 times weaker as an antagonist (Franckowiak et al. 1985). Figure 3 shows the effect of the enantiomers of BAY K 8644 on the monophasic action potential and the isometric force of contraction in an isolated guinea-pig papillary muscle. After a control contraction, 1 μM of the antagonistic (+)-enantiomer was given. This reduced both action potential duration and contractility considerably. An additional 1 μM of (−)-BAY K 8644 antagonized this calcium antagonistic effect and markedly prolonged action potential duration and increased isometric force. Another calcium agonistic DHP, 202-791, has almost identically potent agonistic and antagonistic enantiomers (Hof et al. 1985); therefore the apparently better cardioselectivity (Gross et al. 1990) of the racemic mixture is brought about only by a combination effect.

Economy of Contraction and Safety

Large scale clinical trials with new positive inotropic drugs of the phosphodiesterase (PDE)inhibitors or partial β-adrenergic agonist class have shown deleterious effects on survival in long-term treatment of heart failure patients

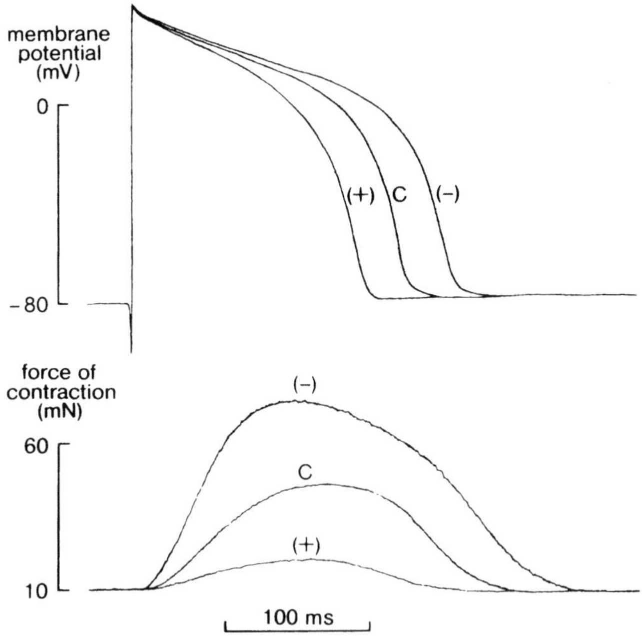

Fig. 3. Effect of the (+)- and the (−)-enantiomers of BAY K 8644 on action potential and force of isometric contraction in an isolated guinea-pig papillary muscle. After a control registration (*C*), first $10^{-6} M$ of the (+)-enantiomer was given. Thereafter $10^{-6} M$ of the (−)-enantiomer were added. (From Franckowiak et al. 1985)

(Yusuf and Teo 1990; Packer et al. 1991; Uretsky et al. 1990; Xamoterol in Severe Heart Failure Study Group 1990). This is most probably mechanism-related and may be due to an overproportionate increase of energy consumption of the heart when stimulated by these cAMP-dependent inotropes. Therefore, the net efficiency of inotropic stimulation by different interventions was compared in isolated working guinea-pig hearts (Gross et al. 1990) (Fig. 4). Gross efficiency, as obtained by dividing pressure-volume work (with the hearts paced at a constant rate) by oxygen consumption, was 11%. This is in good agreement with data reported in the literature (Siess et al. 1981). When the calcium concentration in the perfusate was increased to 2.2 m*M*, stroke work almost doubled. For this inotropic response the net efficiency was 20%. By adjusting the concentration of ouabain, BAY K 8644, isoprenaline, amrinone, or pimobendane, the same increase of cardiac performance was achieved. Interestingly, only with ouabain or BAY K 8644 could the same net efficiency as seen with calcium be achieved, while the stimulation with isoprenaline, amrinone, or pimobendane markedly reduced net efficiency by ⅓–¼; this means that these drugs, acting via cAMP, cause an overproportionate increase of energy consumption even under constant heart rate.

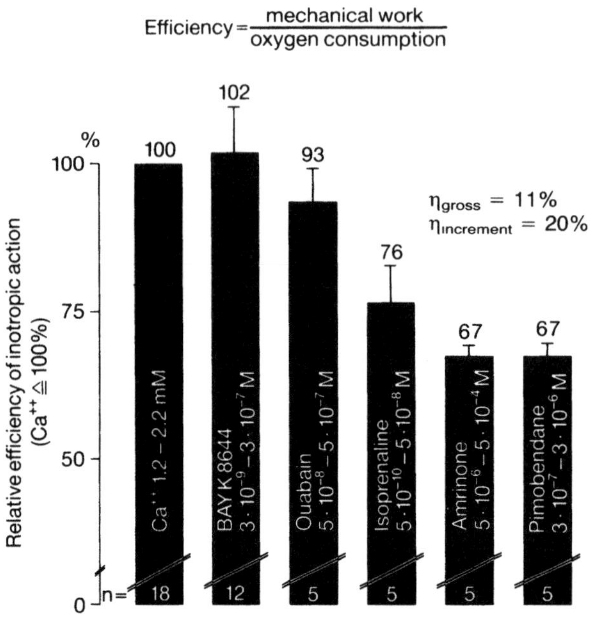

Fig. 4. Net efficiency of the increase of cardiac performance under stimulation with various inotropic drugs. The means with their standard errors are given; *n*, number of experiments. (From Gross et al. 1990)

If this is so in the healthy myocardium, inotropic stimulation of the diseased myocardium, e.g., in the case of secondary heart failure after myocardial infarction, may still bring about an energy deficit. The effect of the calcium agonist BAY K 8644 was therefore tested in isolated working rat hearts which were subjected to low flow hypoxia (Fig. 5). BAY K 8644 (10 n*M*) increased left ventricular $(dP/dt)_{max}$ during normal perfusion by about 35%. When, however, the hearts were made hypoxic by reducing coronary perfusion to about 10% of control flow for 60 min, there was no indication of a positive inotropic effect during the whole hypoxic period. Obviously, the myocytes are still able to quickly switch off their mechanical performance, both with and without the compound, when they become hypoxic. When normal perfusion is restored, recovery of the hearts is even better than under "placebo." From this it becomes evident that there is no reason to consider that this novel positive inotropic principle is "whipping the sick horse to death", since calcium agonists lose their cardiostimulatory effects if the myocytes are in an energetically poor condition. This is also further confirmed by the fact that in isolated perfused guinea-pig hearts the cardiostimulatory effect of BAY K 8644 is relatively low when the hearts are paced at 240 beats/min as compared to the large inotropic effect observed at a pacing rate of 140 beats/min (data not shown). Another observation, in

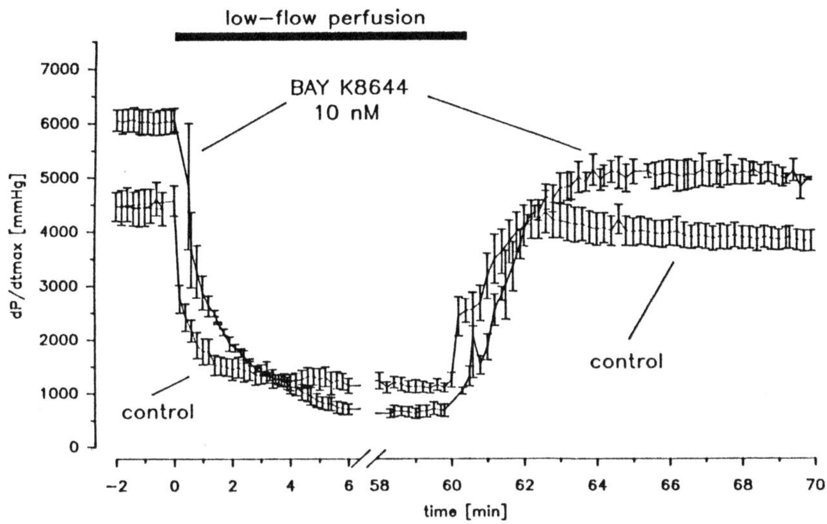

Fig. 5. Effect of 60 min low flow perfusion and reperfusion on left ventricular contractility (measured from dP/dt_{max}) in seven isolated, working rat heart preparations under control conditions and in the presence of 10 n*M* BAY K 8644 throughout the experiment

the Langendorff heart, can be seen in a similar context: At a low (0.6 m*M*) extracellular calcium concentration the positive inotropic effect of BAY K 8644 increases up to very high (300 ng/ml) concentrations, with an IC_{50} of 12 n*M*, whereas under a higher (1.8 m*M*) calcium concentration it begins to decline again above 10 n*M* (data not shown). Therefore, the calcium-induced calcium channel inactivation is still operative under the influence of the calcium agonist.

Mechanism of Action

Calcium channel activation and inactivation were studied in isolated guinea-pig atrial cells (Bechem et al. 1985) using the patch-clamp technique (Hamill et al. 1981). During a depolarizing voltage step (−)-BAY K 8644 causes a concentration-dependent increase of the peak calcium current (Fig. 6). After repolarization the time constant of the "tail-current," reflecting the mean open time of the single channels, is prolonged under the influence of the calcium agonist. At high concentrations the current decays almost monoexponentially, while at lower concentrations the decay is biphasic. This reflects receptor occupancy by the compound; at about the K_D value obtained from binding experiments (Janis et al. 1984) the two components (a fast decay, as under control conditions, and a prolonged time constant, as under high (−)-BAY K 8644-concentrations) are almost equal. This in-

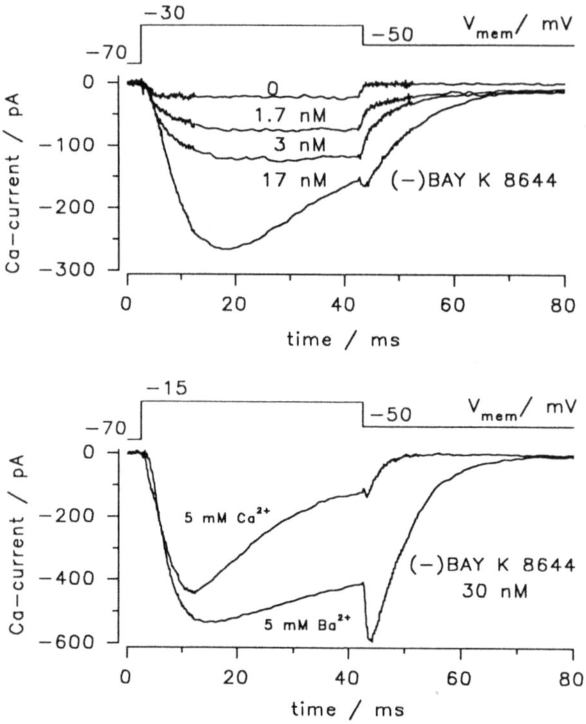

Fig. 6. *Upper panel*, effect of increasing concentrations of (−)-BAY K 8644 on calcium current during a depolarizing step and on "tail currents" after a repolarizing step (clamp protocol at the *top*). *Lower panel*, similar experiment as above, in the presence of 5 m*M* calcium and after replacement by 5 m*M* barium

dicates that under these conditions half of the total number of available calcium channels has bound the compound, while the other half is free. The relative proportion of the two components reflect receptor occupancy.

The hypothesis of the myocyte defending itself against calcium overload under the influence of the agonist is further corroborated by patch-clamp studies: When calcium ions are the charge carriers, a marked inactivation of the calcium current can be seen, which is almost abolished when calcium is replaced by barium ions (Fig. 6).

The schematic model in Fig. 7 tries to explain the mechanism of action of the calcium agonists on the calcium channel: The channel can either be in its resting (closed) state or it can voltage-dependently switch to the open state. The reaction velocities for both directions have the same slope of their voltage-dependence and are given as the open and closed times over membrane potential in the figure inset. The calcium channel binds a calcium agonistic DHP with an association constant of $5 \times 10^6/M/\mathrm{s}$ and a dissociation constant of 0.02/s reflecting a K_D value of 4 n*M*. This drug binding does

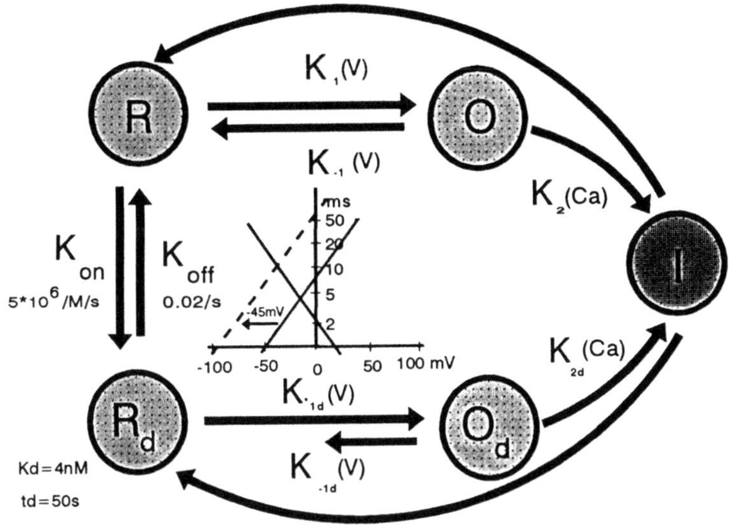

Fig. 7. Reaction scheme for the calcium channel. *R*, resting state; *O*, open state; *I*, inactivated state. The suffix *d* indicates the drug-bound state. The *inset* shows the voltage-dependence of the single channel closed times (*negative slope*) and the open times (*positive slope*). Note that the curve for the open times is shifted by 45 mV to the left (*broken line*) under BAY K 8644

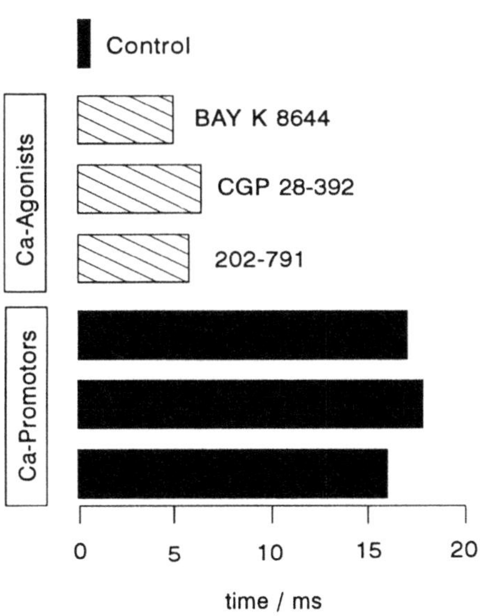

Fig. 8. Mean open times of single calcium channels under control conditions, under the influence of the calcium agonists BAY K 8644, CGP 28-392, 202-791 and three Ca promotors at a membrane potential −50 mV

not change the voltage-dependence of channel opening, but slows down the back-reaction: the voltage-dependence of the open times is shifted in the hyperpolarizing direction by about 45 mV. This results in a higher probability of the channel to be in the open state, the basis for calcium agonism. Since, however, the calcium dependent channel inactivation is not impaired, the probability of the channel to go into the inactivated state is also increased, the basis for calcium antagonism. This may help to understand the dualistic action of DHPs which had already been observed before (Thomas et al. 1984; Sanguinetti and Kass 1984).

Cardioselective Compounds: Ca Promotors

The search for compounds which differ in the balance between calcium agonistic and antagonistic effects has led to DHPs which are cardioselective. In patch-clamp studies, they were found to induce a three times greater prolongation of the mean open times of the calcium channels than the "pure" agonists BAY K 8644, CGP 28-392 (Erne et al. 1984), and 202-791 (Hof et al. 1985) (Fig. 8); hence, they have been named Ca promotors.

The dose-response curve for intravenous injection of such a promotor in anesthetized, spontaneously hypertensive rats (SHRs) (Fig. 9) impressively documents the cardioselctivity: while there is a marked dose-dependent increase of left ventricular $(dP/dt)_{max}$ (as an index of inotropy), from resting values of about 13 000 mm Hg/s up to more than 22 000 mm Hg/s, there is no rise of diastolic blood pressure; rather, there is a tendency to a decrease in conjunction with a small increase in pulse pressure.

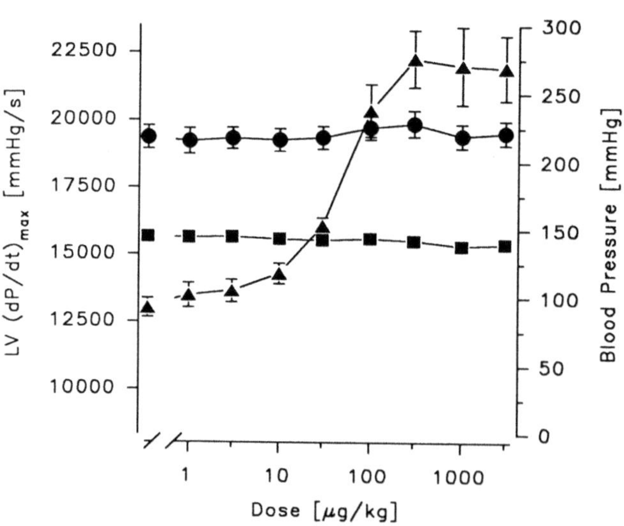

Fig. 9. Dose-response curves for intravenous injection of Ca promotor on left ventricular (dP/dt)max (*triangles*), systolic (*circles*), and diastolic (*squares*) arterial blood pressure in ten spontaneously hypertensive rats. Means ± standard errors

Table 1. Positive inotropic principles

	Glycosides	cAMP-dependent		Calcium promotor
		Catecholamines	PDE inhibitors	
Inotropic effect	Limited (therapeutic index)	Strong (β-receptor down-regulated)	Moderate	Strong, broad range
Vascular effect	Vasoconstricting	Vasodilating	Vasodilating	Vasoneutral
Tolerance development	None	+++	(+)	None
Net efficiency of contraction	100%	<75%	<75%	100%
Effect on heart rate	Decrease	Increase	Moderate increase	No effect or slight decrease
Effect on blood pressure	Slight increase	Decrease	Decrease	No effect

PDE, phosphodiesterase.

In Table 1 the characteristics of the positive inotropic principles used in the treatment of congestive heart failure are compared with those of the Ca promotors: from this it becomes evident that these marked differences are very much in favor of the Ca promotor. If the promising data collected so far in preclinical studies are confirmed in clinical trials, this novel principle may contribute to a better and more efficacious therapy of congestive heart failure. There is certainly a need for it.

References

Bechem M, Pieper F, Pott L (1985) Guinea-pig atrial cardioballs. Basic Res Cardiol 80 [Suppl]:19–22

Bechem M, Hebisch S, Schramm M (1988) Ca-agonists: new sensitive probes for Ca-channels. Trends Pharmacol Sci 9:257–261

Erne P, Bürgisser E, Bühler FR, Dubach B, Kühnis H, Meier M, Rogg H (1984) Enhancement of calcium influx in human platelets by CGP 28-392, a novel dihydropyridine. Biochem Biophys Res Commun 118:842–847

Franckowiak G, Bechem M, Schramm M, Thomas G (1985) The optical isomers of the 1,4-dihydropyridine BAY K 8644 show opposite effects on the Ca-channels. Eur J Pharmacol 114:223–226

Gross R, Bechem M, Kayser M, Schramm M, Taniel R, Thomas G (1985a) Effects of the Ca-agonistic dihydropyridine BAY K 8644 on the heart. In: Fleckenstein A, van Breemen C, Gross R, Hoffmeister F (eds) Cardiovascular effects of dihydropyridine-type calcium antagonists and agonists. Springer, Berlin Heidelberg New York, pp 218–232

Gross R, Kayser M, Schramm M, Taniel R, Thomas G (1985b) Cardiovascular effects of the Ca-agonistic dihydropyridine BAY K 8644 in conscious dogs. Arch Intern Pharmacodyn Ther 277:203–216

Gross R, Bechem M, Hebisch S, Schramm M (1990) Ca-Agonists. In: Abraham S, Amitai G (eds) Calcium channel modulators in heart and scmooth muscle: basic mechanisms and pharmacological aspects. VCH Weinheim/Deerfield Beach Balaban, Rehovot/Philadelphia, pp 353–365

Hamill OP, Marty A, Neher E, Sakmann B, Sigworth FJ (1981) Improved patch-clamp techniques for high-resolution current recording from cells and cell-free membrane pathches. Pflugers Arch 391:85–100

Hof RP, Rüegg UT, Hof A, Vogel A (1985) Stereoselectivity at the calcium channel: opposite action of the enantiomers of a 1,4-dihydropyridine. J Cardiovasc Pharmacol 7:689–693

Hwang KS, van Breemen C (1985) Effects of the agonist BAY K 8644 on ^{45}Ca-influx and net Ca-uptake into rabbit smooth muscle. Eur J Pharmacol 116:299–305

Janis RA, Rampe D, Sarmiento JG, Triggle DJ (1984) Specific binding of the Ca-channel activator BAY K 8644 to membranes from cardiac muscle and brain. Biochem Biophys Res Commun 121:317–323

Packer M, Carver JR, Rodeheffer RJ, Ivanhoe RJ, DiBianco R, Zeldis SM, Hendrix GH, Bommer WJ, Elkayam U, Kukin ML, Mallis GI, Sollano JA, Shannon J, Tandon PK, DeMets DL, for the PROMISE Study Research Group (1991) Effect of oral milrinone on mortality in severe conjestive heart failure. N Engl J Med 325:1468–1475

Sanguinetti MC, Kass RS (1984) Regulation of cardiac calcium channel current and contractile activity by the dihydropyridine BAY K 8644 is voltage-dependent. J Mol Cell Cardiol 16:667–670

Schramm M, Thomas G, Towart R, Franckowiak G (1983) Novel dihydropyridines with positive inotropic action through activation of Ca-channels. Nature 203: 535–537

Schramm M, Towart R, Lamp B, Thomas G (1985) Modulation of calcium ion influx by the 1,4-dihydropyridines nifedipine and BAY K 8644. J Cardiovasc Pharmacol 7:493–496

Siess M, Stieler K, Seifart HJ (1981) Zur Wirkung von ARL-115 BS auf Funktion und Sauerstoffverbrauch isolierter Meerschweinchenherzvorhöfe im Vergleich zu g-Strophantin und Theophyllin. Arzneimittelforschung 31:165–170

Thomas G, Gross R, Schramm M (1984) Calcium channel modulation: ability to inhibit or promote calcium influx resides in the same dihydropyridine molecule. J Cardiovasc Pharmacol 6:1170–1176

Uretsky BF, Jessupo M, Konstam MA, Sandberg A, for the Enoximone multicenter trial group (1990) Multicenter trial of oral enoximone in patients with moderate to moderately severe congestive heart failure. Lack of benefit compared with placebo. Circulation 82:774–780

Vater W, Kroneberg G, Hoffmeister F, Kaller H, Meng K, Oberdorf A, Puls W, Schloßmann K, Stoepel K (1972) Zur Pharmakologie von 4-(2'Nitrophenyl)-2,6-dimethyl-1,4-dihydropyridin-3,5-dicarbon-säuredimethylester (Nifedipin, BAY A 1040). Arzneimittelforschung 22:1–14

Xamoterol In Severe Heart Failure Study Group (1990) Xamoterol in severe heart failure. Lancet 336:1–6

Yusuf S, Teo K (1990) Inotropic agents increase mortality in patients with congestive heart failure. Circulation 82 [Suppl]:673

Nimodipine and Nervous System Function

J. Traber, F.J. van der Staay, and J. de Vry

Nimodipine is a Ca^{2+} antagonist of the 1,4-dihydropyridine type that specifically blocks the L-type Ca^{2+} channel by reducing its opening probability. Binding sites for nimodipine are distinctly located in the central nervous system (CNS), especially in the hippocampal formation and the cortex. These brain structures play an important role in the regulation of cognitive processes. Nimodipine acts not only on neurons but also on glial cells (Hertz et al. 1989). This finding may be highly relevant for nimodipine's action, given the fact that 50% of the cells in the CNS consist of glial cells which support and modulate the function of neurones in the CNS. Finally, there are binding sites for nimodipine on CNS blood vessels which thus provide another target for the drug.

The Calcium Hypothesis

Calcium overload of cells leads to functional disturbances and finally to cell death. This can occur under acute conditions in the range of minutes, hours, or days after stroke or heart failure, but also under chronic conditions, over several months or even years. The Ca^{2+} hypothesis of brain aging states that a moderate increase in intracellular Ca^{2+} over a long period of time may finally cause the same damage as a large increase of intracellular Ca^{2+} during a short period of time (Khatchaturian 1989; Fig. 1). Accordingly, a CNS-specific Ca^{2+} channel blocker like nimodipine should exert interesting pharmacological activity after acute and chronic administration.

Stroke and Nimodipine

Nimodipine not only counteracts the increase in intracellular Ca^{2+} levels but also reduces the extent of cellular damage in the cortical gyrus of cats after ischemic stroke, induced by unilateral occlusion of the middle cerebral

Bayer-Tropon Institute for Neurobiology, Troponwerke, Berliner Strasse 156, 51063 Cologne, Germany

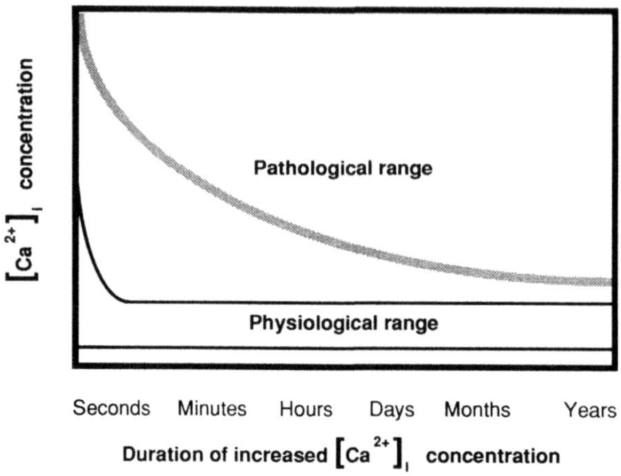

Fig. 1. The calcium hypothesis. A small disturbance of calcium homeostasis, with a sustained increase in intracellular Ca^{2+} over a long period of time, has similar consequences on cellular integrity as those produced by a large increase in intracellular Ca^{2+} over a short period of time. (From Khachaturian 1989)

artery (Uematsu et al. 1989). As another example, nimodipine reduces the infarct size after middle cerebral artery occlusion in the rat (Bielenberg and Beck 1991).

Cognition and Nimodipine

Nimodipine improves learning and memory in a broad range of testing paradigms and in a great variety of species (see also Disterhoft, this volume). In old rats, for example, it improves the acquisition of a simple water maze task (Schuurman and Traber 1989a,b), and it facilitates classical conditioning of the eyeblink response in young and aging rabbits (Deyo et al. 1989). It also improves the retention of a leverpress response in young adult rats (see below). Sandin and colleagues (1990) observed facilitation of recent memory performance in a delayed response paradigm in old rhesus monkeys.

Nimodipine ameliorates dysfunctions which were caused by experimentally induced damage. Nimodipine improved the acquisition of lever pressing on a complex differential reinforcement of low rate responding (DRL) schedule in the Skinner box after bilateral lesioning of the anterior hippocampus (Finger et al. 1990). In a DRL schedule, the interval between two responses must exceed a critical delay. Only responses meeting this criterion are reinforced, whereas all responses with shorter interresponse times are not rewarded. In the study by Finger et al., rats had to learn to suppress a lever press response for at least 20 s. The lesioned nimodipine-treated rats acquired this very complex task as efficiently as the sham-operated rats did.

A newly developed learning and memory task may serve as an example to illustrate the cognition enhancing effects of nimodipine in more detail. The 24-h retention performance of an incompletely acquired bar press response on a continuous reinforcement (CRF: every bar-press is reinforced) schedule was used as the behavioral paradigm to assess cognition enhancing

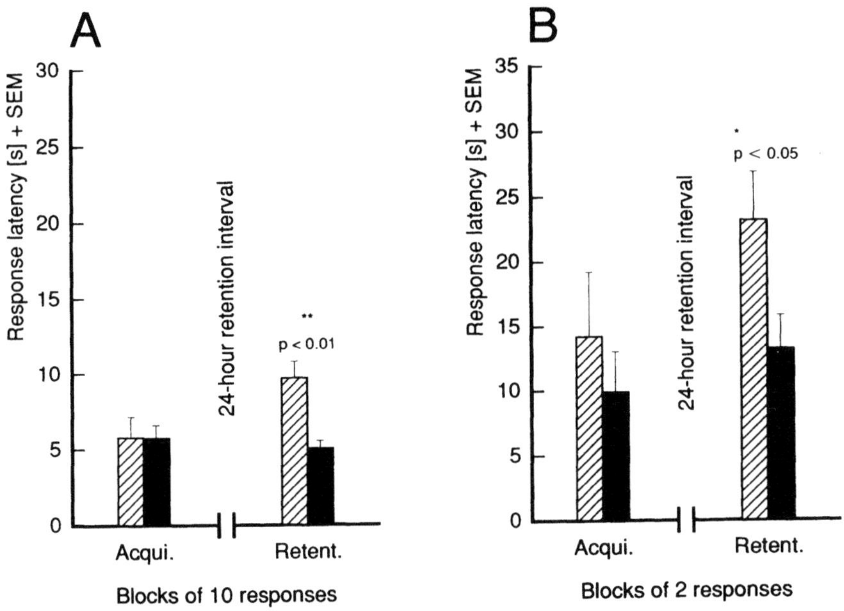

Fig. 2A,B. Effects of a single administration of nimodipine (10 mg/kg, p.o.) on the retention, by young adult Wistar rats, of an incompletely acquired lever press response in an operant conditioning task in a Skinner box. **A** The acquisition session was terminated after 50 lever press responses. **B** Acquisition was terminated after 10 lever press responses. Nimodipine was given orally only once, 30 min before the start of the half hour acquisition session. In **A**, the mean latency of the last ten lever press responses of the acquisition session and of the first ten lever press responses of the retention session are depicted. Analogously, in **B**, the mean latency of the last two lever press responses of the acquisition session and of the first two lever press responses of the retention session are shown. In both studies, nimodipine-treated rats had a better retention performance than control rats, whereas no effects were observed on acquisition. The number of animals per group which acquired the lever press response during the half hour acquisition session was: **A** Control (*hatched columns*), 5 of 10; nimodipine-treated (*blackened columns*) 7 of 10. **B** Control (*hatched columns*), 7 of 10; nimodipine-treated (*blackened columns*), 8 of 10

effects of nimodipine. It was investigated whether a single dose of nimodipine (10 mg/kg, po) given 30 min before the start of a CRF acquisition session would improve retention of the lever press response, measured 24 h later. The acquisition session was terminated when the rat had made 50 lever press responses. In a modified version of the test, acquisition was terminated after ten lever press responses.

Both experiments revealed that nimodipine, given 30 min before the start of the acquisition session, improved performance in the retention session 24 h later, i.e., the bar press latency at the start of the retention session was shorter than that of the untreated control rats (Fig. 2).

The same behavioral paradigm was used to assess whether long-term administration of nimodipine in the diet (1000 ppm) for 4 months would ameliorate retention in aged 24-month-old Wistar rats. Long-term dietary enrichment with nimodipine again appeared to improve retention. Due to the high variability in the performance of aged rats, however, this observation was not confirmed statistically. Thus, the memory enhancing effects of nimodipine were confirmed, using young adult rats, whereas a trend to ameliorate memory performance was seen in aged rats treated over a prolonged period with nimodipine.

Motor Functions and Nerve Conductance Velocity

It has consistently been shown that long-term dietary nimodipine treatment (800–1000 ppm) is able to retard the age-related decrease of motor functions in rats. In a typical experiment, treatment started when the rats were 24 months old and lasted for 4 months. Under these conditions, the footprint patterns of nimodipine-treated rats were similar to those of young ones and were virtually free of the abnormal patterns shown by the untreated control rats (Gispen et al. 1988; Schuurman and Traber 1989a,b; Schuurman et al. 1987; van der Zee et al. 1990). This finding might have significance for the clinical administration of nimodipine, as clear antidegenerative effects of long-term treatment were found. In an attempt to further elucidate the mechanism for this antidegenerative effect, the nerve conductance velocity of the sciatic and caudal nerves of nimodipine-treated and matched, untreated, aged rats was measured (van der Zee et al. 1990). Nimodipine treatment consisted of 800 ppm in the food for 20 weeks starting when the rats were 24 months old. In untreated rats, nerve conductance velocity decreased with age. Nimodipine treatment partially prevented this decrease and increased nerve conductance velocity even in rats with existing disturbances at the start of treatment. An alternative approach to study the antidegenerative and neuroprotective effects consists of assessing the effects of nimodipine in animals with experimentally induced deficiencies. After a crush lesion of the sciatic nerve, the walking patterns of rats are severely disturbed. Slow spontaneous recovery of the walking pattern occurs afterwards. Nimodipine accelerated the functional recovery in this model (van der Zee et al. 1987; Gispen et al. 1988).

Nimodipine and Diabetes Neuropathy

A single streptozotocin injection induces diabetes mellitus in rats. The animals develop a diabetic neuropathy in which the nerve conductance velocity in peripheral sensory and motor nerves is reliably decreased. During 10 weeks, diabetic rats were treated, i.p. with nimodipine (20 mg/kg) every 48 h, and nerve conductance velocity was measured every 2 weeks. Nimodipine significantly counteracted the diabetes-induced decrease in nerve conductance velocity in a preventive fashion (Kappelle et al. 1992). Even more interestingly, nimodipine also ameliorated the signs of an existing neuropathy in streptozotocin-induced diabetic rats (Kappelle et al. 1993).

Effects of Nimodipine on the Cerebrovascular System

Originally, Kazda and colleagues (1982) showed that nimodipine affects the cerebrovascular system. In primates, for example, nimodipine enhanced cerebral blood flow without influencing cerebral metabolism (Harper et al. 1981).

During aging, a number of perivascular malformations appear in the rat brain, such as microvascular fibrosis, membranous inclusions, and basement membrane thickenings (de Jong et al. 1991). In one experiment, 24-month-old rats received either placebo or nimodipine-enriched food for half a year. Nimodipine treatment reduced the occurrence of perivascular fibrotic deposits in their brains (de Jong et al. 1990, 1992). The most effective dose appeared to be 850 ppm. Whether these effects on the microvessels might provide a morphological basis for the improvement of cognitive and sensorimotor functions seen in aged rats after long-term dietary nimodipine treatment remains to be elucidated.

AIDS Dementia and Parkinson Dementia

Dreyer and colleagues (1990) found that the AIDS virus surface protein gp120, after binding to retinal ganglion cells and hippocampal neurons in culture, dramatically increased intracellular Ca^{2+} levels, eventually leading to cell death. This increase could dose-dependently be prevented by nimodipine. They suggested that the Ca^{2+} increase may, at least in part, be responsible for some signs of AIDS-induced dementia and that nimodipine could be of value in its treatment.

Nimodipine and Depression

The rat and the mouse forced swimming test has been used for the detection of anti-depressant drugs (Porsolt et al. 1977, 1978). In this test model, a rodent is put into a glass container filled with water. After some vigorous attempts to escape, the animal realizes the impossibility to leave and "gives up" by just floating on the surface of the water. Different kinds of antidepressant drugs reduce the immobility, which can be taken as a measure of potential antidepressive activity. Interestingly, nimodipine is able to reduce the immobility. Figure 3 shows the effect of oral administration of 3, 10, and 30 mg/kg nimodipine in a rat forced swimming test. Nimodipine reduced the immobility at a dose of 10 mg/kg, suggesting that the compound might be a useful antidepressant with a low margin of side effects. A similar antidepressant-like effect of nimodipine has been suggested by Czyrak and colleagues (1990).

Nimodipine and Addiction

There is experimental evidence that Ca^{2+} channel antagonists (e.g., nifedipine: Engel et al. 1988; verapamil: Rezvani and Janowsky 1990; Goe

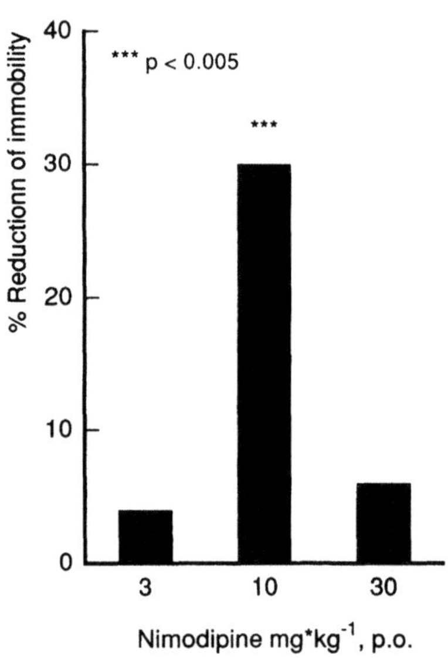

Fig. 3. Antidepressive effect of nimodipine in the rat forced swimming test. Rats ($n = 6$ per group) were given a 20 min swimming trial on day 1. Nimodipine was given orally in a dose of 3, 10, or 30 mg/kg, 23, 5, and 1 h before a 5 min swimming test on day 2. The percentage reduction of immobility, compared with a vehicle pretreated control group, in the 10 mg group reflects antidepressive properties of the compound

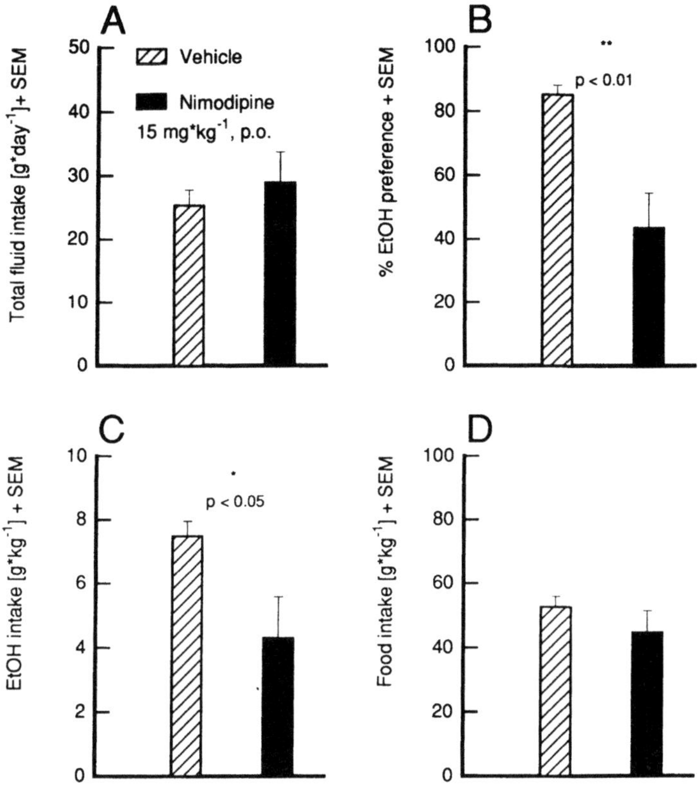

Fig. 4A–D. Selective alcohol (*EtOH*) preference reducing effects of nimodipine in ALKO alcohol accepting (AA) rats. Rats showing a clear preference for EtOH (10%) over water in a two bottle preference test were treated orally 5 min before an 18 h test session. The effects of nimodipine on **A** total fluid intake (EtOH + water), **B** % EtOH preference, **C** EtOH intake, and **D** food intake are depicted

5438: Pucilowski et al. 1992) suppress ethanol consumption in rats. In order to test the effect of nimodipine in a free choice paradigm, we used ALKO alcohol accepting rats (AA rats). This line of rats was selected from the Sprague Dawley strain for its preference to drink a 10% ethanol solution rather than water (Ritz et al. 1989). Preliminary results show that nimodipine potently and dose-dependently suppresses alcohol preference in these rats (Fig. 4), i.e., they then prefer to drink water. Unexpectedly, the Ca^{2+} channel agonist BAY K 8644 also suppresses alcohol preference. Thus, it is questionable whether these effects are due to the Ca^{2+} channel antagonistic activity of nimodipine.

A study by Whittington and colleagues (1991) showed that long-term dihydropyridine treatment (either nitrendipine or nimodipine) prevented the occurrence of the ethanol withdrawal syndrome in mice following long-term treatment with ethanol. Nimodipine has also been found to suppress intravenous self-administration of cocaine and morphine in mice in a dose-dependent manner (the ED_{50} being 14.5 and 11.4 mg/kg for cocaine and morphine, respectively; Kuzmin et al. 1992).

Conclusion

Nimodipine clearly improves nervous system function after short- and long-term administration in a great variety of models. Thus, the compound not only reduces brain infarction after experimental stroke but also evidently improves age-related dysfunctions (cognition, motor functions) and displays antidegenerative and regenerative effects (crush lesions, neuropathies). In addition, antidepressive and anticraving activity has been characterized in animal models. Nimodipine and other Ca^{2+} channel blockers may therefore have an interesting potential in the treatment of a broad range of nervous system diseases.

References

Bielenberg GW, Beck T (1991) The effects of dizocilpine (MK-801), phencyclidine, and nimodipine on infarct size 48 h after middle cerebral artery occlusion in the rat. Brain Res 552:338–342

Czyrak A, Mogilnicka E, Siwanowicz J, Maj J (1990) Some behavioral effects of repeated administration of calcium channel antagonists. Pharmacol Biochem Behav 35:557–560

de Jong GI, de Weerd H, Schuurman T, Traber J, Luiten PGM (1990) Microvascular changes in aged rat forebrain. Effects of chronic nimodipine treatment. Neurobiol Aging 11:381–389

de Jong GI, Jansen ASP, Horváth E, Gispen WH, Luiten PGM (1991) Nimodipine effects on cerebral microvessels and sciatic nerve in aging rats. Neurobiol Aging 13:73–81

de Jong GI, Nyakas C, Schuurman T, Luiten PGM (1992) Aging-related alterations in behavioral activation and cerebrovascular integrity in rats are dose-dependently influenced by nimodipine. Neurosci Res Commun 12:1–8

Deyo RA, Straube KT, Disterhoft JH (1989) Nimodipine facilitates associative learning in aging rabbits. Science 243:809–811

Dreyer EB, Kaiser PK, Offermann JT, Lipton SA (1990) HIV-1 coat protein neurotoxicity prevented by calcium channel antagonists. Science 248:364–367

Engel JA, Fahlke C, Hulthe P, Hard E, Johannessen K, Snape B, Svensson L (1988) Biochemical and behavioral evidence for an interaction between ethanol and calcium channel antagonists. J Neural Transm 74:181–193

Finger S, Green L, Tarnoff ME, Mortman KD, Andersen A (1990) Nimodipine enhances new learning after hippocampal damage. Exp Neurol 109:279–285

Gispen WH, Schuurman T, Traber J (1988) Nimodipine and neural plasticity in the peripheral nervous system of adult and aged rats. In: Morad M, Nayler W,

Kazda S, Schramm M (eds) The calcium channel: structure, function and implications. Springer, Berlin Heidelberg New York, pp 491–502

Harper AM, Craigen L, Kazda S (1981) Effect of the calcium antagonist, nimodipine, on cerebral blood flow and metabolism in the primate. J Cereb Blood Flow Metab 1:349–356

Hertz L, Bender AS, Woodbury DM, White HS (1989) Potassium-stimulated calcium uptake in astrocytes and its potent inhibition by nimodipine. J Neurosci Res 22:209–215

Kappelle AC, Bravenboer B, Traber J, Erkelens DW, Gispen WH (1992) The Ca^{2+} antagonist nimodipine counteracts the onset of an experimental neuropathy in streptozotocin induced, diabetic rats. Neurosci Res Commun 10:95–104

Kappelle AC, Bravenboer B, van Buren T, Traber J, Erkelens DW, Gispen WH (1993) Amelioration by the Ca^{2+} antagonist nimodipine of an existing neuropathy in the streptozotocin-induced, diabetic rat. Br J Pharmacol 108:780–785

Kazda S, Garthoff B, Krause HP, Schloßmann K (1982) Cerebrovascular effects of the calcium antagonist dihydropyridine derivative nimodipine in animal experiments. Arzneimittelforschung 32:331–338

Khatchaturian ZS (1989) The role of calcium regulation in brain aging: reexamination of a hypothesis. Aging 1:17–34

Kuzmin A, Zvartau E, Gessa GL, Martellotta MC, Fratta W (1992) Calcium antagonists isradipine and nimodipine suppress cocaine and morphine intravenous self-administration in drug-naive mice. Pharmacol Biochem Behav 41:497–500

Porsolt RD, LePichon M, Jalfre M (1977) Depression: a new animal model sensitive to antidepressant treatment. Nature 266:730–732

Porsolt RD, Anton G, Blavet M, Jalfre M (1978) Behavioural despair in rats, a new model sensitive to antidepressant treatments. Eur J Pharmacol 47:379–391

Pucilowski O, Rezvani AH, Janowsky DS (1992) Suppression of alcohol and saccharin preference in rats by a novel Ca^{2+} channel inhibitor, Goe 5438. Psychopharmacology 107:447–452

Rezvani AH, Janowsky DS (1990) Decreased alcohol consumption by verapamil in alcohol preferring rats. Prog Neuropsychopharmacol Biol Psychiatry 14:623–631

Ritz M, George FR, Meisch RA (1989) Ethanol self-administration in ALKO rats: I. Effects of selection and concentration. Alcohol 6:227–233

Sandin M, Jasmin S, LeVere TE (1990) Aging and cognition: facilitation of recent memory in aged nonhuman primates by nimodipine. Neurobiol Aging 11:573–575

Schuurman T, Traber J (1989a) Old rats as an animal model for senile dementia: behavioral effects of nimodipine. In: Bergener M, Reisberg B (eds) Diagnosis and treatment of senile dementia. Springer, Berlin Heidelberg New York, pp 295–307

Schuurman T, Traber J (1989b) Effects of nimodipine on behavior of old rats. In: Traber J, Gispen WH (eds) Nimodipine and central nervous system function: new vistas. Schattauer, Stuttgart, pp 195–208

Schuurman T, Klein H, Beneke M, Traber J (1987) Nimodipine and motor deficits in aged rats. Neurosci Res Commun 1:9–15

Uematsu D, Greenberg JH, Hickey WF, Reivich M (1989) Nimodipine attenuates both increase in cytosolic free calcium and histologic damage following focal cerebral ischemia and reperfusion in cats. Stroke 20:1531–1537

van der Zee CEEM, Schuurman T, Traber J, Gispen WH (1987) Oral administration of nimodipine accelerates functional recovery following peripheral nerve damage in the rat. Neurosci Lett 83:143–148
van der Zee CEEM, Schuurman T, Gerritsen van der Hoop R, Traber J, Gispen WH (1990) Beneficial effect of nimodipine on peripheral nerve function in aged rats. Neurobiol Aging 11:451–456
Whittington MA, Dolin SJ, Patch TL, Siarey RJ, Butterworth AR, Little HJ (1991) Chronic dihydropyridine treatment can reverse the behavioural consequences of and prevent adaptation to, chronic ethanol treatment. Br J Pharmacol 103:1669–1676

Nimodipine and Learning in Aging Rabbits

J.F. Disterhoft, J.R. Moyer, Jr., L.T. Thompson, and M. Kowalska

Abstract

A major focus of our research has been to describe how neuronal excitability is changed during learning in the young adult brain and how neurons in the aging brain may be impaired in their ability to produce such changes. In our approach we have utilized eyeblink conditioning and the in vivo and in vitro rabbit hippocampus for behavioral, neurophysiological, and biophysical studies of associative learning. We have also investigated the potential contribution of nimodipine in enhancing learning in aging subjects, with a focus on the role of calcium-mediated processes in learning. The hippocampus is known to be important for learning and memory consolidation and to be profoundly affected by aging and Alzheimer's disease. Hippocampal ablation was shown to block acquisition and/or extinction in eyeblink tasks, with effects most prominent in trace conditioning. Extracellular recordings in vivo have demonstrated increased excitability of hippocampal neurons to the conditioned stimulus in eyeblink conditioning. Experiments in our laboratory indicated that this increased excitability resulted from a conditioning-specific reduction in the post-burst afterhyperpolarization (AHP) of CA1 neurons in hippocampal slices. The AHP is a postsynaptic response regulating neuronal excitability and is generated by an outward calcium-dependent potassium current. This hyperpolarizing response is increased in aging hippocampal neurons, presumably as a result of increased intracellular calcium levels in aging neurons. Consequently, aging neurons are less able to increase their excitability and thus show adaptive change during associative learning. The calcium channel blocker nimodipine facilitated acquisition of trace eyeblink conditioning in the aging rabbit. Convergent data suggest that this learning enhancement may also be mediated by changes in hippocampal neuronal excitability. Nimodipine apparently increases excitability by reducing calcium influx through voltage-gated calcium channels, with a secondary reduction in the post-burst AHP. The relevance of our findings to potential clinical applications in aging and/or in Alzheimer's disease is discussed.

Dept. of Cell Molecular and Structural (CMS) Biology, Northwestern University Medical School, 303 E. Chicago Avenue, Chicago, IL 60611-3008, USA

Introduction

The neurobiological substrates of associative learning in mammalian brain are complex and incompletely understood. As is the case with the study of substrates of learning and plasticity in invertebrates, considerable progress has been made in recent years (Alkon 1984; Thompson 1990). One approach has been to adopt the use of a "model behavioral system" to analyze learning mechanisms (Woodruff-Pak and Thompson 1985). Learning tasks which are impaired in human amnesics, such as delayed matching to sample and complex list learning, have been used in subhuman primates to demonstrate the involvement of the hippocampus and related temporal lobe structures in transferring information from immediate (short-term) to more permanent (long-term) storage (Squire 1987; Squire and Zola-Morgan 1991). We have adopted eyeblink conditioning in the rabbit as a relatively simple behavioral model of associative learning which is quite amenable to analysis (Akase et al. 1989; Gormezano 1986; Thompson et al. 1992a). Because of our interest in the involvement of the hippocampus and temporal lobe structures in this task, we have concentrated on trace eyeblink conditioning in our recent work. In the trace conditioning task, rabbits are given a short duration tone conditioned stimulus (CS) followed by a corneal airpuff unconditioned stimulus (US) with a blank 500 ms "trace" period intervening, during which they must maintain a representation of the tone in order to anticipate and reduce the impact of the US. Successful acquisition of this task in the rabbit depends upon an intact hippocampus (Moyer et al. 1990; Solomon et al. 1986). The eyeblink conditioning task was originally developed in the human and was later adapted for the rabbit by Gormezano (1966). In some of our recent experiments, we have been exploring the comparability of eyeblink conditioning in the aging rabbit and aging human in more detail (Disterhoft et al. 1991b; Carrillo et al. 1993).

Hippocampal multiple and single neurons are involved in eyeblink conditioning in large numbers (Akase et al. 1988). Hippocampal CA1 and CA3 pyramidal neurons show a striking tendency to form a temporal model of the eyeblink conditioned response. Changes in their averaged firing rates anticipate the behavioral response both in terms of appearance during the overall learning process and on individual training trials (Akase et al. 1988; Berger et al. 1983). We have examined CA1 pyramidal neurons in hippocampal slices prepared from conditioned rabbits and have observed a striking reduction in the post-burst afterhyperpolarization (AHP) after learning (de Jonge et al. 1990). This reduction, which would make the neurons more excitable and/or capable of firing multiple action potentials to previously subthreshold excitatory inputs, is likely to be a major contributor to the enhanced firing to the conditioned stimulus which we and others have observed as learning proceeds (Disterhoft et al. 1986). It is interesting that the AHP is generated by a calcium-mediated outward potassium current, and thus regulated by intracellular calcium levels.

The connection between our systems and cellular analyses of eyeblink conditioning and the effects of dihydropyridines on learning in aging animals is straightforward. First, we know that the hippocampus suffers many important neural alterations which are correlated with learning deficits in aging subjects (Barnes 1983; Decker 1987; Geinisman et al. 1986). This is particularly true of the devastating consequences of Alzheimer's disease and its correlated severe learning and memory impairments. The formation of plaques and tangles during Alzheimer's disease is associated with deterioration in the afferents to and the efferents from the hippocampus and of the primary pyramidal neurons of the hippocampus proper (van Hoesen and Hyman 1990). At about the same time as we initially reported that the slow AHP is reduced in hippocampal neurons from young rabbits after learning, Landfield and Pitler (1984) reported that the AHP duration is prolonged in CA1 pyramidal neurons from aging rats. They suggested that this alteration in the AHP response could underlie some of the learning deficits seen during the aging process. Their report was consistent with the so-called calcium hypothesis of aging, which posits that excess intracellular calcium in neurons, as well as other cells in the body, may play a causal role in the deterioration of some functions which occurs during aging (Khachaturian 1989; Landfield 1987).

Second, we know that eyeblink conditioning in both aging rabbits and humans is impaired in comparison to that observed in young individuals (Deyo et al. 1989; Disterhoft et al. 1991b; Graves and Solomon 1985; Woodruff-Pak et al. 1987). We hypothesized that this aging deficit could be related to decreased excitability of hippocampal neurons. Reduced excitability could be caused by an increase in the amplitude or duration of the post-burst slow AHP, resulting in a reduced capacity to process information in the hippocampal system. The question that we posed was whether we could reverse some of the deficits in learning ability in the aging animal with a pharmacological agent which had the potential to reduce or reverse the aging-specific enhanced slow AHP. Preliminary data were available prior to our studies from human clinical trials which were brought to our attention by Dr. Ronald Janis. When the dihydropyridine nimodipine was used as a treatment for subarachnoid hemorrhage, it was suggested that this compound enhanced learning ability in aging human patients in addition to and apart from its effect on recovery from stroke (Bono et al. 1985).

Nimodipine, an L-type calcium channel antagonist, can readily cross the blood-brain barrier (van den Kerckhoff and Drewes 1989), so it should have good direct access to hippocampal neurons. In our first series of experiments, we decided to evaluate the effects of nimodipine on learning in aging rabbits. We administered nimodipine via indwelling intravenous catheters to young or aging rabbits and evaluated its effects on trace eyeblink conditioning (Deyo et al. 1989). The striking finding was that nimodipine enhanced learning in this hippocampally dependent task in aging animals. In fact, they learned at the same rate or slightly faster than young rabbits given either vehicle alone or nimodipine. This finding was subsequently replicated and extended using oral doses of nimodipine (Deyo et al. 1989; Straube et al. 1990).

Our observation of nimodipine's behavioral facilitation was an exciting one, although it clearly raised many questions for us to pursue. In the remainder of this chapter we will summarize our progress addressing some of these open questions. Specifically, what is the dose-response relationship to the behavioral effect? Can we make a determination of nimodipine serum levels necessary to enhance behavioral learning? Does nimodipine increase neuronal excitability selectively in aging brain in the awake rabbit? If so, is this excitability increase mediated by effects on the calcium-dependent AHP? Does nimodipine antagonize calcium influx directly in aging neurons? As will be seen, these questions are interrelated. The answers to them appear to show that excess calcium influx is associated with learning deficits in the aging rabbit.

Dose-Response Studies

In our initial report, nimodipine enhanced hippocampally dependent trace eyeblink conditioning in aging rabbits when given intravenously at a dose of 1 μg/kg/min (Deyo et al. 1989). This dose had no effect on learning rate

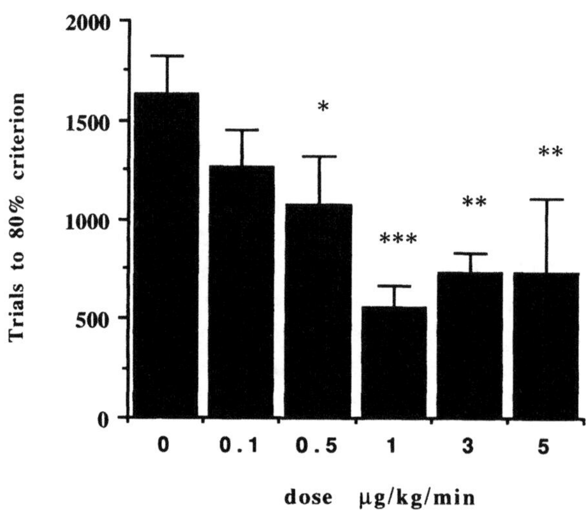

Fig. 1. Nimodipine doses greater than 0.5 μg/kg/min facilitated acquisition of 500 ms trace eyeblink conditioning in aging rabbits. The mean (±SEM) number of trials required to reach a behavioral criterion of 80% conditioned responses is shown. *Asterisks* indicate significance level of post-hoc Fisher's comparison of the drug group from the vehicle control group: $^{*}p < 0.05$, $^{**}p < 0.01$, $^{***}p < 0.001$. The behavioral effects of doses of 0.5 μg/kg/min or greater were not significantly different between groups. (Adapted from Kowalska and Disterhoft 1992)

in young rabbits. We have now determined the relationship between intravenous dose of nimodipine administered and learning rate and the relationship between nimodipine serum concentration and learning rate in aging rabbits (Kowalska and Disterhoft 1992).

The experimental procedures used were similar to those previously reported (Deyo et al. 1989). Nimodipine was given to aging (>36 months) rabbits in various doses via intravenous catheters during the daily training sessions. Nimodipine was suspended in a vehicle containing polyethylene glycol, alcohol, and water. The 500 ms trace eyeblink conditioning paradigm was used for training. The doses of nimodipine tested were 0.1, 0.5, 1.0, 3.0, or 5.0 μg/kg/min. A comparable volume of vehicle was used for the controls. Aging rabbits which received a daily dose of nimodipine 0.5 μg/kg/min or greater required fewer trials to reach a behavioral criterion of 80% conditioned responses than control animals (Fig. 1).

When training was completed, blood samples were taken and serum levels of nimodipine were determined (Krol et al. 1984). In general, all serum concentrations above 10 ng/ml were correlated with enhanced learning rates. Serum levels above this dose offered no significant behavioral advantages. The serum concentrations measured ranged from nondetectable in control subjects (and/or nonlearning rabbits) to over 500 ng/ml in rabbits that learned.

Nimodipine Effects on Hippocampal Activity In Vivo

Given that nimodipine facilitated acquisition of trace eyeblink conditioning in aging rabbits and that trace eyeblink conditioning is dependent upon the hippocampus, we wished to determine the effects of nimodipine administration on hippocampal neuronal activity. Evidence for selective enhancement of excitability of hippocampal neuronal activity in aging as compared to young rabbits would be consistent with the behavioral effects observed and reviewed above.

Rabbits were prepared as for eyeblink conditioning with the addition of the implantation of a chronic moveable microdrive which allowed a bundle of ten microwires to be passed through the CA1 hippocampus (Kubie 1984). Drug administration was via a chronically implanted intravenous catheter. Several observations were made (Thompson et al. 1990) which can be summarized briefly (Fig. 2). The administration of nimodipine caused an enhancement of CA1 pyramidal neuron basal firing rate which was rapid in onset and offset. Altered activity occurred within 20 min after intravenous nimodipine administration and rapidly returned to basal rates after drug administration ceased. Neuronal activity was enhanced in vivo at concentrations of nimodipine above 0.1 μg/kg/min. The dose which caused the maximal enhancement of firing rate was 1 μg/kg/min, the dose which was initially shown to facilitate eyeblink conditioning in the aging rabbit (Deyo

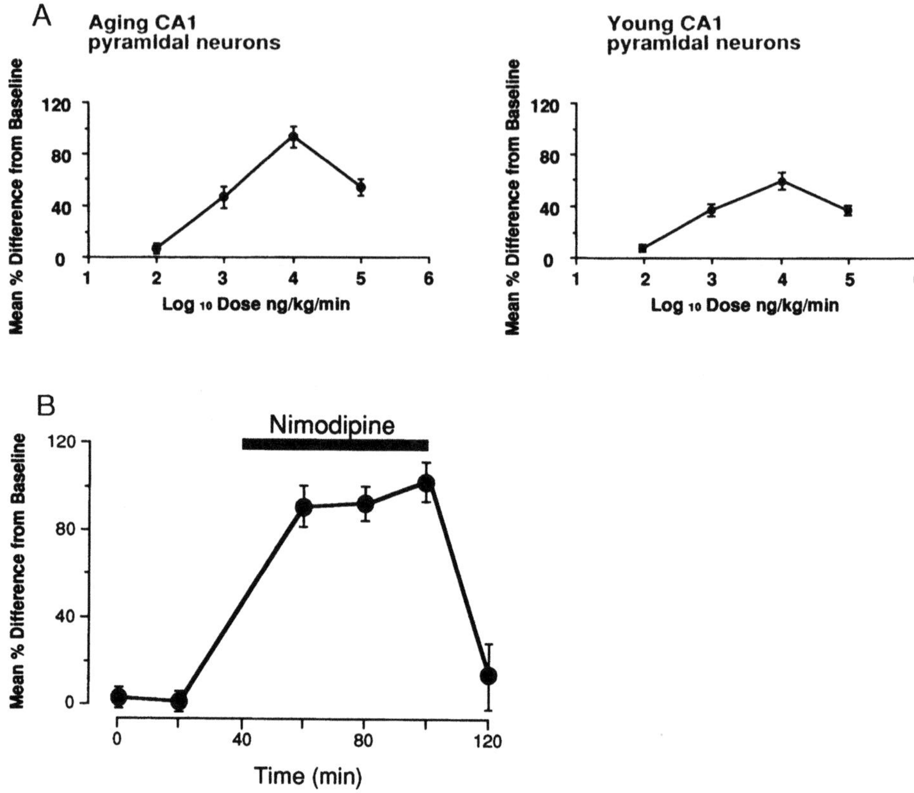

Fig. 2A–B. Intravenous nimodipine given to awake rabbits dose-dependently enhanced the basal firing rates of hippocampal pyramidal cells. **A** Doses above 100 ng/kg/min significantly increased basal firing in both age groups. However, nimodipine enhanced neuronal firing in aging rabbits to a significantly greater degree than in young rabbits. **B** The effects of nimodipine were fairly rapid both in onset and in offset. As seen at a dose of 1 μg/kg/min, maximal effects were seen within 20 min of the start of intravenous infusion and persisted throughout drug application. The observed increase in excitability had ended within 20 min of the termination of infusion. (Adapted from Thompson et al. 1990)

et al. 1989). Finally, the effect of nimodipine application was considerably larger in aging than in young rabbits. Additional data not summarized here demonstrated that the firing rate enhancement was not seen in CA1 pyramidal neurons when nifedipine, flunarizine, or vehicle was administered. The fact that nifedipine was not effective is likely due to its relatively limited ability to cross the blood-brain barrier (van den Kerckhoff and Drewes 1989). It is clear that nimodipine enhances cerebral blood flow in the rabbit (Haws and Heistad 1984). The fact that flunarizine had no effect on hippocampal pyramidal cell firing rates suggests that the nimodipine effects are not due solely to an enhancement of cerebral blood flow. A broad range of flunarizine concentrations were used, some of which should have been sufficient to increase cerebral blood flow. We have interpreted our in vivo neuronal recording data to suggest that the enhancement of hippocampal neuron firing reflects a direct action of nimodipine on these neurons. Of course, such an interpretation is difficult to prove in vivo. Therefore, we have addressed this question with neurophysiological analyses using the in vitro brain slice preparation.

Nimodipine Effects on the Calcium-Activated Afterhyperpolarization In Vitro

Hippocampal pyramidal cells, and many other neuron types, possess slow calcium-activated outward potassium currents (Hotson and Prince 1980; Lancaster and Adams 1986; Schwindt et al. 1992). These currents are activated by the calcium influx into the neurons during action potentials, which occur either singly or in bursts. These potassium currents are considered to be important modulators of overall firing rates of neurons, since they largely determine the membrane resting potential in the periods between action potentials (Storm 1990). As such, it is interesting to note that the slow AHP often lasts for relatively long periods (seconds) after a burst of action potentials, and is acted on by modulatory neurotransmitters such as acetylcholine and norepinephrine (Cole and Nicoll 1983; Madison and Nicoll 1986). We have been very interested in the slow AHP, since our initial observation that associative learning is related to a reduction in this after potential in CA1 hippocampal pyramidal neurons (Disterhoft et al. 1986). The reduction in the slow AHP observed after eyeblink conditioning is learning-specific (Disterhoft et al. 1988), occurs in CA1 pyramidal neurons and not dentate granule neurons (de Jonge et al. 1990), and is localized by the slice preparation both within the hippocampus, and further within the postsynaptic neuron because it is demonstrable in the absence of sodium-dependent neurotransmission (Coulter et al. 1989; Disterhoft et al. 1986). A reduction in the slow AHP during and after eyeblink conditioning could be a major membrane-level mechanism for enhanced excitability of CA1 neurons. Evidence for this increased excitability is seen in the fact that a large percentage of single CA1 neurons show enhanced firing rates to the CS during and after training, with a temporal pattern which precedes and mimics the developing eyeblink conditioned response (Berger et al. 1983).

The slow afterhyperpolarization was initially shown by Landfield and Pitler (1984) to be of longer duration in CA1 neurons from aging rats. They suggested that this increase, which would make CA1 neurons less excitable, would impair the use of hippocampal circuitry to form new memories in aging animals. When we examined the slow AHP in CA1 neurons in hippocampal slices prepared from aging (>36 month) rabbits, we observed that

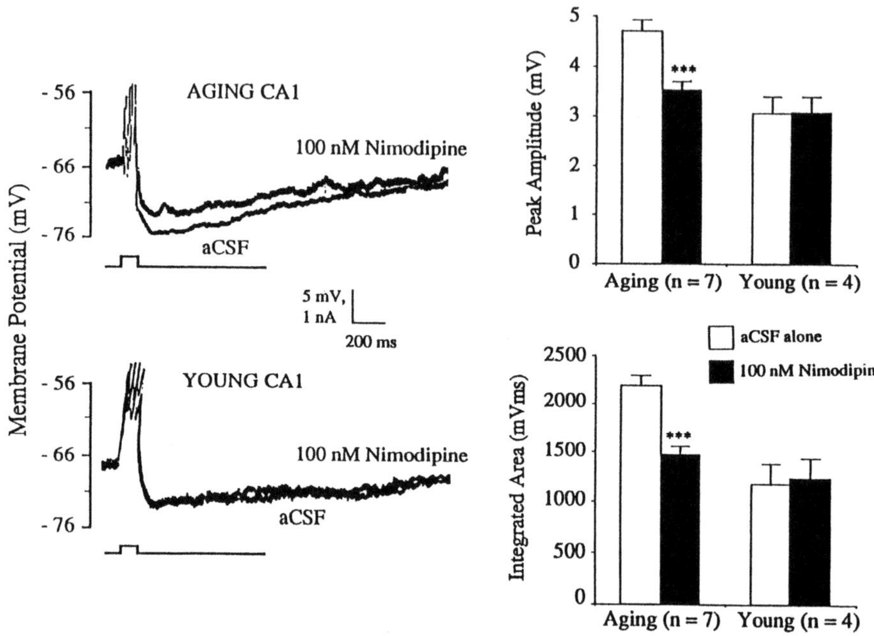

Fig. 3. Nimodipine at a concentration of 100 n*M* produced a significant reduction in the postburst afterhyperpolarization (AHP) of CA1 neurons in slices from aging but not young rabbits. The reduction was present both in the integrated area of the AHP (a measure of duration) and in the peak amplitude of the response. Scale in *left panel*, 5 mV, 1 nA and 200 ms. (Adapted from Moyer et al. 1992)

the AHP was considerably larger both in amplitude and in total area, representing an enhancement of the AHP which lasting for more than 800 ms in aging neurons (Moyer et al. 1992; compare aging and young controls in Fig. 3). As further evidence for the reduced excitability, aging CA1 neurons also showed considerably more spike frequency accommodation to a long depolarizing pulse than did cells from younger rabbits. Previous investigators have pointed out a relationship between the AHP and accommodation (Madison and Nicoll 1984). If the AHP is large, the neuron reduces its firing rate to a long depolarizing pulse more rapidly (i.e., the cell shows more accommodation).

Our interest was next to determine what effect calcium channel antagonists have on this enhanced calcium-dependent potential in aging neurons. When the dihydropyridine calcium channel blocker nimodipine was added to the bathing solution at high concentrations (10 μM), both the AHP and accommodation were reduced in young and aging neurons (Moyer et al. 1992). When more physiologically reasonable concentrations were used, a striking differential effect was observed between aging and young neurons.

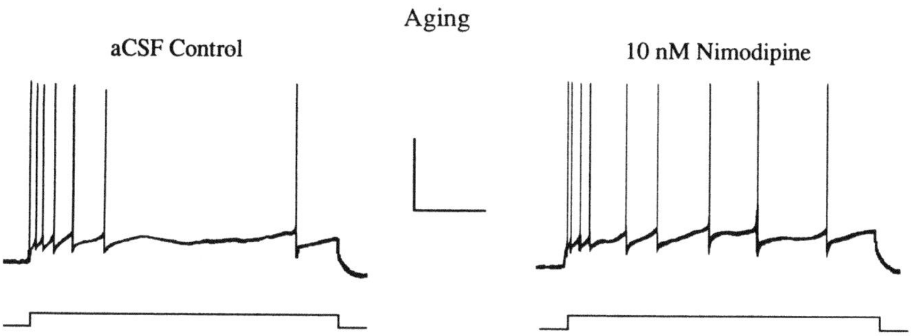

Fig. 4. Nanomolar concentrations of nimodipine decreased accommodation in aging neurons. *Left panel* shows accommodation of an aging neuron to a prolonged depolarizing current injection before nimodipine. *Right panel* shows the same aging neuron after bath application of 10 n*M* nimodipine. In aging neurons ($n = 4$), nimodipine significantly increased the number of action potentials elicited during the accommodation pulse ($F(1,1) = 14.027$, $p < 0.01$). Scale: 40 mV, 2 nA and 200 ms. (Adapted from Moyer et al. 1992)

At concentrations as low as 100 n*M*, nimodipine reduced the amplitude and duration of the slow AHP in aging but not in young neurons (Moyer et al. 1992; Fig. 3). It is interesting to note that nimodipine reduced the AHP into the same range as that observed in young neurons. The effects of nimodipine on spike frequency accommodation were similar. High concentrations of nimodipine reduced accommodation in both young and aging neurons. However, nimodipine in concentrations as low as 10 n*M* were effective in reducing spike frequency accommodation in aging CA1 neurons (Moyer et al. 1992; Fig. 4), while concentrations below 1.0 μ*M* were ineffective on young cells.

These effects were not limited to nimodipine. We observed comparable effects using nifedipine concentrations of 10 μ*M* on both the slow afterhyperpolarization and accommodation. Although we did not do a systematic examination of nifedipine's effects at lower concentrations, our results suggest that when nifedipine has direct access to neurons as in the in vitro preparation, nifedipine effectively modulated calcium-mediated potassium currents and their consequences.

Nimodipine Effects on the Calcium Action Potential

The experiments reviewed above clearly demonstrate that nimodipine, in physiologically meaningful concentrations, increased excitability of hippocampal neurons in aging brain by reducing the calcium-activated outward potassium current which underlies the post-burst AHP. These data raise the question whether nimodipine acts directly on the calcium action potential, directly on the potassium hyperpolarizing potential, or on the intervening intracellular processes between calcium influx and the activation of the outward potassium current. To begin to address these issues, we have done a series of experiments examining the effect of nimodipine on the calcium action potential of CA1 pyramidal neurons from young and aging hippocampal slices (Moyer and Disterhoft 1993).

Hippocampal slices were prepared according to our usual procedures. Neurons were recorded with cesium chloride-filled microelectrodes to block outward potassium currents. Following the isolation of a CA1 pyramidal neuron, excitatory synaptic potentials were evoked by stimulation of the Schaffer collaterals. Then $4\,\mu M$ tetrodotoxin was added to the bathing solution to block sodium-dependent neurotransmission, as evidenced by the lack of synaptic potentials evoked via the excitatory Schaffer collateral inputs.

First, we noted that the calcium action potential was larger in aging CA1 pyramidal neurons. More specifically, the initial fast phase of the action potential was relatively unchanged in aging neurons while the slower, plateau phase was both larger in amplitude and longer in duration in aging than in young CA1 neurons (Fig. 5). Since the slow AHP is dependent upon calcium influx for its activation, the enhancement of the slow calcium action potential is completely appropriate as a substrate for enhancement of the slow AHP (Fig. 3). These data are consistent with previous reports of enhanced calcium action potentials in CA1 (Pitler and Landfield 1990) neurons from aging rats.

Application of nimodipine had effects which were rather similar to those previously observed in the AHP studies. Nimodipine at high concentrations ($10\,\mu M$) reduced the plateau phase of the calcium action potential of both

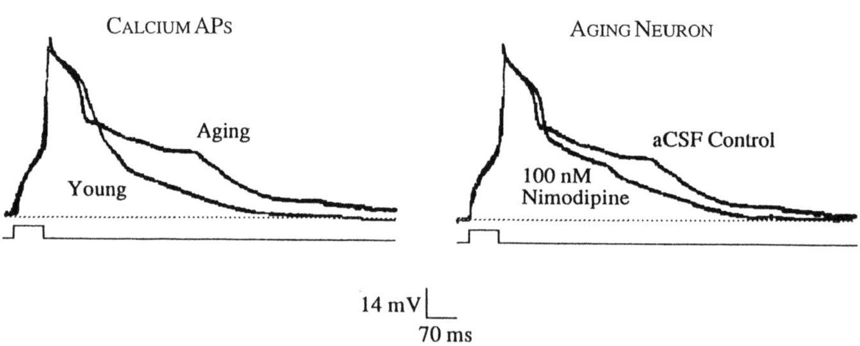

Fig. 5. The slow plateau phase of calcium action potentials of aging CA1 pyramidal neurons were enhanced in both amplitude and duration as compared to those of young neurons. Relatively low concentrations of nimodipine ($100\,nM$) reduced the amplitude and duration of this plateau phase in aging but not young neurons. After nimodipine treatment, calcium influx in aging neurons was returned to levels closely approximating those of young neurons. (Adapted from Moyer and Disterhoft 1993)

young and aging CA1 neurons, with a greater effect seen in aging neurons. As with the AHP, differential effects were observed when lower concentrations of nimodipine were evaluated. The plateau phase of the calcium action potential was reduced only in aging neurons by application of nimodipine at concentrations as low as 100 n*M* (Fig. 5). Figure 5 demonstrates clearly that the portion of the calcium action potential which is effected by nimodipine is the plateau phase. Thus, a significant portion of the enhanced calcium influx observed in aging neurons is selectively blocked by nimodipine.

Comments and Conclusions

The series of studies discussed here investigated the role of the hippocampal formation in associative learning, particularly in trace eyeblink conditioning. We have demonstrated that in this model system hippocampal activity is both related to and required for successful acquisition. We and others have shown that hippocampal neurons fire vigorously in a pattern that mimics the conditioned response during development of and after learning of this task. We have demonstrated that a calcium-activated outward potassium conductance, which underlies the post-burst AHP, is reduced in hippocampal neurons from conditioned animals. This cellular change appears to be a major contributor to the enhanced excitability that these neurons demonstrate after learning. This same conductance is conversely increased in hippocampal neurons from aging rabbits, which makes these neurons less excitable, and could underlie the observed learning deficits in aging animals.

The question that we next posed was quite straightforward. Could we use a pharmacological compound (such as nimodipine) effective at blocking calcium influx in other preparations to enhance learning rates in aging rabbits? If so, could we demonstrate neurophysioloical data in the intact aging rabbit and biophysical data in the in vitro slice that support our hypothesized mechanism of action, i.e., blockade of L-type voltage-dependent calcium currents in hippocampal neurons? The experiments summarized here answered these questions in the affirmative.

Nimodipine facilitated learning of a hippocampally dependent task in aging rabbits. Nimodipine seems to have no effect on learning this paradigm in young animals, although we have not investigated this thoroughly. As mentioned above, we interpret our data within the context of the calcium hypothesis of aging. Nimodipine seems to be effective in aging brains because it reduces the elevated intracellular calcium levels in these cells, at least in a temporary fashion. It is interesting to note that aging particularly affects the hippocampus, when measured either neurophysiologically (Barnes 1983; Barnes et al. 1987; Lamour et al. 1987; Moyer et al. 1992) or neuroanatomically (Decker 1987; Geinisman et al. 1986; Mani et al. 1986). We have summarized a series of neurophysiological studies which suggest that one of nimodipine's actions in the rabbit is to enhance hippocampal neuronal excitability. A number of behavioral studies done in recent years have shown positive behavioral effects of nimodipine in aging primates or rats using behavioral measures dependent upon the hippocampus for their successful acquisition (Sandin et al. 1990). Those studies which have used young animals have been concerned with recovery from brain damage and have demonstrated that nimodipine facilitates such recovery (Finger et al. 1990; LeVere et al. 1989). Since large brain lesions may lead to excess calcium levels in neurons throughout the brain, these studies may have a considerable amount in common with our work on aging animals. Convergent lines of evidence thus suggest that nimodipine is especially useful in compensating for functional loss in compromised brain tissue. Since both aging and lesions may cause excess calcium influx, nimodipine's direct actions as a neuronal calcium channel antagonist are beneficial in both conditions.

Nimodipine effects on calcium currents at high concentrations was reported previously in single electrode voltage studies by Landfield (1989). An effect on aging neurons and a differential effect on aging neurons at physiological concentrations of nimodipine had not previously been reported. Although we did not directly test the effect of agents which interact with other types of calcium channels, nimodipine reversed the majority of the enhanced calcium action potential seen in aging neurons. Therefore, our data suggest strongly that the late plateau portion of the calcium action potential which is increased in aging neurons is mediated primarily by increased L-type voltage-sensitive calcium conductances. We noted above that there is a temporal convergence in the alterations which occur in both the calcium action potential and in the slow AHP. It is quite conceivable that the enhanced AHP in aging CA1 neurons is dependent upon an increased plateau phase of the calcium action potential. Further experiments are required and should shed further light on the mechanism of aging-related changes in calcium action potentials. Our experiments demonstrate that physiologically reasonable concentrations of nimodipine can modulate aging related changes and bring cells back into the range of slow AHP and calcium action potential amplitude shown by hippocampal neurons from young animals.

Our behavioral and psychopharmacological data from our rabbit model system parallel observations made in humans. Aging humans (mean age 65 years) showed impaired acquisition of 500 ms trace eyeblink conditioning as compared to young adults (mean age 25 years; Disterhoft et al. 1991b). In both species, impairments are significant by middle age (30 months for rabbits; 40 years for humans). Eyeblink conditioning tasks do not require use of nonmnemonic cognitive capacities that also decline with aging, including visuospatial coordination, language and list processing. Eyeblink conditioning is impaired in subjects with temporal lobe dysfunction (Daum et al. 1991) and in Alzheimer's patients, a group with known hippocampal degeneration (Finkbiner and Woodruff-Pak 1991). Our rabbit model system both allows us to evaluate mechanisms of learning deficits occurring in aging humans (including Alzheimer's patients) and to test therapeutic interventions in aging populations. For example, we have nearly completed a clinical trial testing the effects of nimodipine on eyeblink conditioning, as well as on other cognitive and mnemonic tasks, in normal young adult and aging subjects. Similar designs parallel to our animal studies are in progress or planned for patients with Alzheimer's disease or age-associated memory impairments. Promising results from our European colleagues (Baumel et al. 1989; Fischhof et al. 1989; Schmage et al. 1989) suggest that nimodipine should prove efficacious in alleviating some of the learning deficits we have observed in our own work with human subjects.

Our research program combining cellular and subcellular observations with behavioral analyses of associative learning has proven useful for understanding some of the neurobiological alterations underlying aging-associated learning deficits (Disterhoft et al. 1992; Thompson et al. 1992). Our data indicate a significant involvement of calcium influx via L-type voltage-dependent channels in aging-associated biophysical changes in hippocampal neurons. A number of questions remain to be explored, including possible alterations in channel expression, gating and turnover, or changes in genomic transcription or posttranslational modifications of the channel protein or its dihydropyridine binding site. Possible alterations in gating kinetics of calcium-dependent potassium currents in aging neurons (Moyer et al. 1992) also remain to be explored. With increasingly sophisticated analyses using our animal model system, we should be able to optimize development and testing of pharmacological agents to revitalize learning abilities in humans throughout the lifespan.

References

Akase E, Deyo RA, Disterhoft JF (1989) Activity of single hippocampal CA1 pyramidal neurons during trace eye-blink conditioning. Soc Neurosci Abstr 14:394

Alkon DL (1984) Calcium-mediated reduction of ionic currents. A biophysical memory trace. Science 226:1037–1045

Barnes CA (1983) The physiology of the senescent hippocampus. In: Siefert W (ed) Neurobiology of the hippocampus. Academic, London, pp 87–108

Barnes CA, Rao G, McNaughton BL (1987) Increased electrotonic coupling in aged rat hippocampus: a possible mechanism for cellular excitability changes. J Comp Neurol 259:549–558

Baumel B, Eisner LS, Karukin M, MacNamara R, Raphan H (1989) Nimodipine in the treatment of Alzheimer's Disease. In: Bergener M, Reisberg B (eds) Diagnosis and treatment of senile dementia. Springer, Berlin Heidelberg New York, pp 366–373

Berger TW, Rinaldi PC, Weisz DJ, Thompson RF (1983) Single-unit analysis of different hippocampal cells types during classical conditioning of rabbit nictitating membrane response. J Neurophysiol 50:1197–1219
Bono G, Sinforiani E, Trucco M, Cavallini A, Acuto GC, Nappi G (1985) Nimodipine in cCVD patients: Clinical and neuropsychological results of a double-blind crossover study. In: Betz E, Deck K, Hoffmeister F (eds) Nimodipine, pharmacological and clinical properties, Schattauer, Stuttgart, pp 275–287
Carrillo MC, Thompson LT, Naughton BJ, Gabrieli N, Disterhoft JF (1993) Aging impairs trace eyeblink conditioning in humans independent of changes in the unconditioned response. Soc Neurosci Abstr 19: in press
Cole AE, Nicoll RA (1983) Acetylcholine mediates a slow synaptic potential in hippocampal pyramidal cells. Science 221:1299–1301
Coulter DA, Lo Turco JJ, Kubota M, Disterhoft JF, Moore JW, Alkon DL (1989) Classical conditioning reduces amplitude and duration of calcium-dependent afterhyperpolarization in rabbit hippocampal pyramidal cells. J Neurophysiol 61:971–981
Daum I, Channon S, Polkey CE, Gray JA (1991) Classical conditioning after temporal lobe lesions in man: impairment in conditional discrimination. Behav Neurosci 105:396–408
Decker MW (1987) The effects of aging on hippocampal and cortical projections of the forebrain cholinergic system. Brain Res Rev 12:423–438
de Jonge MC, Black J, Deyo RA, Disterhoft JF (1990) Learning-induced afterhyperpolarization reductions in hippocampus are specific for cell type and potassium conductance. Exp Brain Res 80:456–462
Deyo RA, Straube KT, Disterhoft JF (1989) Nimodipine facilitates trace conditioning of the eyeblink response in aging rabbits. Science 243:809–811
Disterhoft JF, Coulter DA, Alkon DL (1986) Conditioning-specific membrane changes of rabbit hippocampal neurons measured in vitro. Proc Nat Acad Sci USA 83:2722–2737
Disterhoft JF, Golden DT, Read HR, Coulter DA, Alkon DL (1988) AHP reductions in rabbit hippocampal neurons during conditioning are correlated with acquisition of the learned response. Brain Res 462:118–125
Disterhoft JF, Black J, Moyer JR Jr, Thompson LT (1991a) Calcium-mediated changes in hippocampal neurons and learning. Brain Res Rev 16:193–220
Disterhoft JF, Conroy SW, Thompson LT, Naughton BJ, Gabrieli JDE (1991b) Age affects eyeblink conditioning and response discrimination in humans. Soc Neurosci Abstr 17:476
Disterhoft JF, Deyo RA, Thompson LT (1992) Nimodipine improves learning and sensorimotor behaviors in aging mammals. In: Meyer EM (ed) The treatment of dementias: a new generation of progress. Plenum, New York, pp 227–240
Finger S, Green L, Tarnoff ME, Mortman KD, Andersen A (1990) Nimodipine enhances new learning after hippocampal damage. Exp Neurol 109:279–285
Finkbiner RG, Woodruff-Pak DS (1991) Classical eyeblink conditioning in adulthood: effects of age and interstimulus interstimulus interval on acquisition in the trace paradigm. Psychol Aging 6:109–117
Fischhof PK, Wagner G, Littschauer L, Rüther E, Apecechea M, Hiersemenzel R, Röhmel J, Hoffmeister F, Schmage N (1989) Therapeutic results with nimodipine

in primary degenerative dementia and multi-infarct dementia. In: Bergener M, Reisberg B (eds) Diagnosis and treatment of senile dementia. Springer, Berlin Heidelberg New York, pp 350–359
Geinisman Y, De Toledo-Morrell L, Morrell F (1986) Loss of perforated synapses in the dentate gyrus: morphological substrate of memory deficit in aged rats. Proc Natl Acad Sci USA 83:3027–3031
Gormezano I (1986) Classical conditioning. In: Sidowski JB (ed) Experimental methods and instrumentation in psychology. McGraw-Hill, New York, pp 385–420
Gormezano I, Prokasy WF, Thompson RF (eds) (1987) Classical conditioning. Lawrence Erlbaum Associates, Hillsdale
Graves CA, Solomon PR (1985) Age-related disruption of trace but not delay classical conditioning of the rabbit's nictitating membrane response. Behav Neurosci 99:88–96
Haws CW, Heistad DD (1984) Effects of nimodipine on cerebral vasoconstrictor responses. Am J Physiol 247:H170–H176
Hotson JR, Prince DA (1980) A calcium-activated hyperpolarization follows repetitive firing in hippocampal neurons. J Neurophysiol 43:409–419
Kachaturian ZS (1989) The role of calcium regulation in brain aging: reexamination of a hypothesis. Aging 1:17–34
Kowalska M, Disterhoft JF (1992) Dose dependent effect of nimodipine on learning rate in aging rabbits. Soc Neurosci Abstr 18:1435
Krol GJ, Noe AJ, Yeh SC (1984) Gas and liquid chromatographic analyses of nimodipine calcium antagonist in blood plasma and cerebrospinal fluid. J Chromatogr 305:105–118
Kubic JL (1984) A driveable bundle of microwires for collecting single-unit data from freely moving rats. Physiol Behav 32:115–118
Lamour Y, Dutar P, Jobert A (1987) Septo-hippocampal neurons: altered properties in the aged rat. Brain Res 416:277–282
Lancaster B, Adams PR (1986) Calcium-dependent current generating the afterhyperpolarization of hippocampal neurons. J Neurophysiol 55:1268–1282
Landfield PW (1987) Increased calcium-current hypothesis of brain aging. Neurobiol Aging 8:346–347
Landfield PW (1989) Nimodipine modulation of aging-related increases in hippocampal calcium currents. In: Traber J, Gispen WH (eds) Nimodipine and central nervous system function. Schattauer, Stuttgart, pp 35–49
Landfield PW, Pitler TA (1984) Prolonged Ca^{2+}-dependent afterhyperpolarizations in hippocampal neurons of aged rats. Science 226:1089–1092
LeVere TE, Brugler T, Sandin M, Gray-Silva S (1989) Recovery of function after brain damage: facilitation by the calcium entry blocker nimodipine. Behav Neurosci 103:561–565
Madison DV, Nicoll RA (1984) Control of repetitive discharge of rat CA1 pyramidal neurones in vitro. J Physiol (Lond) 354:319–331
Madison DV, Nicoll RA (1986) Actions of noradrenaline recorded intracellularly in rat hippocampal CA1 pyramidal neurons, in vitro. J Physiol (Lond) 372:221–244
Mani RB, Lohr JB, Jeste DV (1986) Hippocampal pyramidal cells and aging in the human: a quantitative study of neuronal loss in sectors CA1 to CA4. Exp Neurol 94:29–40

Moyer JR Jr, Deyo RA, Disterhoft JF (1990) Hippocampectomy disrupts trace eyeblink conditioning in rabbits. Behav Neurosci 104:243–252

Moyer JR Jr, Thompson LT, Black J, Disterhoft JF (1992) Nimodipine increases excitability of rabbit CA1 pyramidal neurons in an age- and concentration-dependent manner. J Neurophysiol 68:2100–2109

Moyer JR Jr, Disterhoft JF (1993) Nimodipine decreases calcium action potentials in rabbit hippocampal. CAI neurons in an age- and concentration-dependent manner. Hippocampus (in press)

Pitler TA, Landfield PW (1990) Aging-related prolongation of calcium spike duration in rat hippocampal slice neurons. Brain Res 508:1–6

Sandin M, Jasmin S, LeVere TE (1990) Aging and cognition: facilitation of recent memory in aged nonhuman primates by nimodipine. Neurobiol Aging 11:567–571

Schmage N, Boehme K, Dycka J, Schmitz H (1989) Nimodipine for psychogeriatric use: methods, strategies and considerations based on experience with clinical trials. In: Bergener M, Reisberg B (eds) Diagnosis and treatment of senile dementia. Springer, Berlin Heidelberg New York, pp 374–381

Schwindt PC, Spain WJ, Crill WE (1992) Calcium-dependent potassium currents in neurons from cat sensorimotor cortex. J Neurophysiol 67:216–226

Scoville WB, Milner B (1957) Loss of recent memory after bilateral hippocampal lesions. J Neurol Neurosurg Psychiatry 20:11–21

Scriabine A, Battye R, Hoffmeister F, Kazda S, Towart R, Garthoff B, Schlüter G, Rämsch KD, Scherling D (1985) Nimodipine. In: Scriabine A (ed) New drugs annual: cardiovascular drugs, vol 3. Raven, New York, pp 197–218

Solomon PR, vander Schaff EV, Thompson RF, Weisz DJ (1986) Hippocampus and trace conditioning of the rabbit's classically conditioned nictitating membrane response. Behav Neurosci 100:729–744

Squire L (Ed) (1987) Memory and brain. Oxford, New York

Squire LR, Zola-Morgan S (1991) The medial temporal lobe memory system. Science 253:1380–1386

Storm JF (1990) Potassium currents in hippocampal pyramidal cells. Prog Brain Res 83:161–187

Straube KT, Deyo RA, Moyer JR Jr, Disterhoft JF (1990) Dietary nimodipine improves associative learning in aging rabbits. Neurobiol Aging 11:659–661

Thompson RF (1990) Neural mechanisms of classical conditioning in mammals. Phil Trans R Soc Lond B 329:161–170

Thompson LT, Disterhoft JF, Deyo RA (1990) Nimodipine enhances spontaneous activity of hippocampal pyramidal cells in aging rabbits at a dose that facilitates learning. Brain Res 535:19–130

Thompson LT, Moskal JR, Disterhoft JF (1992a) Hippocampus-dependent learning facilitated by a monoclonal antibody or d-cycloserine. Nature 359:638–641

Thompson LT, Moyer JR Jr, Disterhoft JF (1992b) Cellular mechanisms for nimodipine's reduction of aging-related learning deficits. In: Meyer EM (ed) The treatment of dementias: a new generation of progress. Plenum, New York, pp 241–256

van den Kerckhoff W, Drewes LR (1989) Transfer of nimodipine and another calcium antagonist across the blood-brain barrier and their regional distribution in vivo. In: Bergener WB, Reisberg B (eds) Diagnosis and treatment of senile dementia. Springer, Berlin Heidelberg New York, pp 308–321 van Hoesen GW, Hyman BT (1990) Hippocampal formation: anatomy and the patterns of pathology in Alzheimer's disease. Prog Brain Res 83:445–457

Woodruff-Pak DS, Thompson RF (1985) Classical conditioning of the eyelid response in rabbits as a model system for the study of brain mechanisms of learning and memory in aging. Exp Aging Res 11:109–122

Woodruff-Pak DS, Lavond DG, Logan CG, Thompson RF (1987) Classical conditioning in 3-, 30-, and 45-month-old rabbits: behavioral learning and hippocampal unit activity. Neurobiol Aging 8:101–108

Molecular Biology of Calcium Channels

P. Spreyer[1], J.K. Franz[1], A. Eller[1], P. Rae[1,2], and A. Unterbeck[1,2]

Introduction

Voltage-operated calcium channels (VOCCs) are membrane-spanning multisubunit protein complexes which are the major element controlling calcium entry from the extracellular space into the cytoplasm of excitable cells. VOCCs are predominantly expressed in neuronal and endocrine cells, and in cardiac, smooth, and skeletal muscle.

As voltage-dependent functional units, these calcium pores play an important role in the maintenance of cellular calcium homoeostasis (Kennedy 1989). Further, they are key factors in the control of muscle contraction, the release of neurotransmitters and hormones (Tsien 1983; Hess 1990), the modulation of other ion channels (Marty 1989), and the regulation of transcription (Morgan and Curran 1989; Sheng and Greenberg 1990).

The skeletal muscle calcium channel was the first to be characterized at the molecular level (Tanabe et al. 1987). It is composed of five polypeptides designated alpha-1, alpha-2, beta, gamma, and delta (Fig. 1; Campbell et al. 1988). The alpha-1 subunit (α_1), which contains four domains of six membrane-spanning helices each, forms the calcium pore and is considered to be the subunit that confers voltage sensitivity to the channel complex. The four accessory subunits (α_2, β, γ, and δ) support the structural and functional properties of the channel. While the γ subunit seems to be limited to skeletal muscle, the α_1, α_2, β, and δ subunits are standard components of VOCCs that are also found in other excitable tissues.

Voltage-operated calcium channels were originally classified according to their electrophysiological and pharmacological properties (Bean 1989; Tsien et al. 1991). Low voltage channels, called *T-type* channels, require relatively low membrane potentials for activation, whereas high threshold channels (L, N, and P types) activate at greater positive membrane potentials. The function of *L-type* channels is modulated by three distinct classes of calcium channel ligands (Catterall and Striessnig 1992): dihydropyridines

[1] Bayer AG, Institute for Cardiovascular and Atherosclerosis Research, 42096 Wuppertal, Germany
[2] Present address: Miles Research Center, West Haven, CT 06516, USA

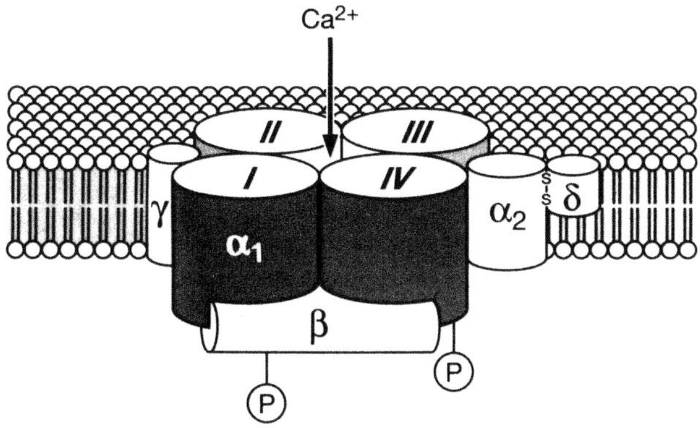

Fig. 1. Subunit composition of voltage-operated calcium channels. α_1, α_2, β, γ, and δ designate calcium channel subunits as described in the text. The α_2 and δ subunits are likely to be linked by disulfide bridges (*SS*). The α_1 and β subunits contain phosphorylation sites (*P*) on the intracellular side of the plasma membrane

(DHPs), phenylalkylamines (PAAs), and benzothiazepines. In contrast, *N-type* and *P-type* channels are insensitive to DHPs. Rather, they are specifically blocked by ω-conotoxin GVIA (Cruz and Olivera 1986) and the funnel web spider toxin ω-Aga-IVA (Mintz et al. 1992), respectively. A compound that specifically blocks *T-type* channels has not yet been identified.

Because of their key role in many important physiological processes, VOCCs present a major target for drug development. In particular, cardiovascular diseases and disorders of the nervous system are areas of intense research activities aimed at identifying novel calcium channel agonists and antagonists. Several compounds modulating calcium flux are already available for clinical use.

Molecular analyses have revealed an unexpected diversity of calcium channels (Perez-Reyes et al. 1990; Snutch et al. 1990). The genes coding for different isoforms of a calcium channel subunit show both high degrees of homology and a complex tissue specific expression pattern. Pharmacological studies of individual channel complexes have thus been constrained by the unavailability of cell lines or tissues which express only one particular type of VOCC. However, molecular biology techniques offer new opportunities to clone cDNAs coding for specific calcium channels and to then display a single channel type at high abundance on the surface of mammalian host cells transfected to express the channel of interest de novo. Molecular cloning and expression of cell type-specific calcium channel subunits thereby provide an innovative and powerful tool for creating drug screening systems that allow in vitro identification of highly selective channel ligands.

The α_1 Subunit

Over the past few years, a number of complete α_1 subunit cDNA clones have been isolated from different species and from a variety of cell lines and tissues, including skeletal, cardiac, and smooth muscle, brain, neuroendocrine glands, and fibroblasts. Nucleotide sequence differences among these cDNAs point to a diversity of Ca^{2+} channels, with the deduced amino acid sequences of all these cDNAs being 30%–70% homologous to one another, and representing proteins with molecular masses of 212–273 kDa.

Based on hydropathy analysis, the primary amino acid sequences of the α_1 subunit polypeptides predict four homologous domains (domains I–IV in Fig. 2), each containing six transmembrane segments. This topology is similiar to that of other voltage operated ion channels (Noda et al. 1984; Kamb et al. 1987). Every third or fourth residue in the fourth transmembrane segment of each domain (S4) is positively charged, and S4 is thus thought to be the voltage sensor of the molecule (Stühmer et al. 1989). The loop between transmembrane segments 5 and 6 in each domain was assumed to be extracellular, but is now believed to fold into the membrane, forming a part of the ion pore and contributing to ion selectivity (Guy and Conti 1990; Heinemann et al. 1992).

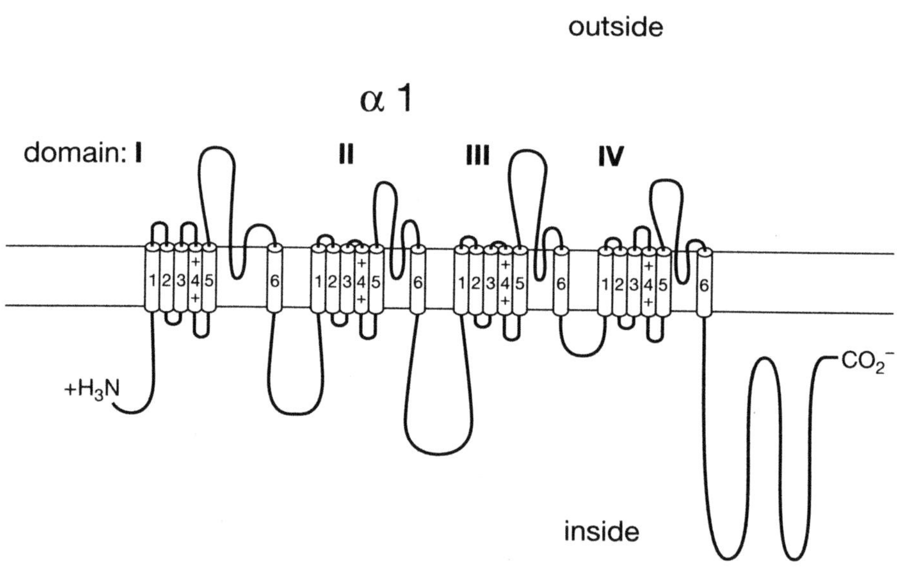

Fig. 2. Linear transmembrane topology of the α_1 subunit of voltage-operated calcium channels as deduced from amino acid hydropathy analysis. Each transmembrane domain (*I–IV*) is composed of six membrane-spanning helices (*1–6*). The fourth helix (*4*) of each domain (*I–IV*) represents the putative voltage-sensor (*+*). (Taken with permission from Catterall and Striessing 1992)

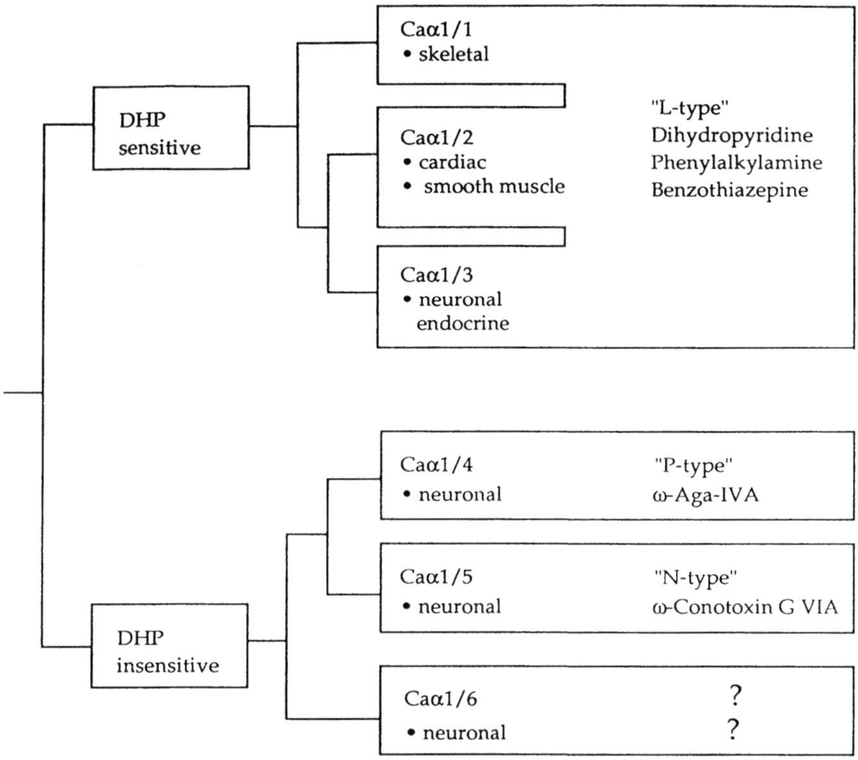

Fig. 3. Putative evolutionary tree of DHP-sensitive and -insensitive α_1 subunits of voltage-operated calcium channels based on amino acid sequence homologies among the gene products Caα_1/1-Caα_1/6

Each of the α_1 subunit cDNAs cloned so far is a transcript of one or another of six different genes (Caα_1/1–6, Fig. 3). From consideration of degrees of amino acid sequence homology among the different α_1 subunits, as well as of pharmacological and electrophysiological data, these genes can be aligned in two major groups: those which encode DHP-sensitive α_1 subunits, represented by Caα_1/1–3; and those coding for DHP-insensitive ones, i.e., Caα_1/4–6.

Genes coding for DHP-sensitive α_1 subunits are expressed in skeletal (Tanabe et al. 1987; Grabner et al. 1991), cardiac (Mikami et al. 1989; Diebold et al. 1992) and smooth muscle (Biel et al. 1990; Koch et al. 1990), and neuroendocrine cells (Seino et al. 1992), in fibroblasts (Soldatov 1992), and in the central nervous system (Hui et al. 1991; Williams et al. 1992a; Snutch et al. 1991).

The skeletal muscle-specific α_1 subunit (Caα_1/1) occurs in two distinct isoforms. The major from is 190 kDa in size and comprises more than 90%

of the Caα_1/1 protein in skeletal muscle; it is a post-translational proteolytic cleavage product of the minor form, a 212 kDa polypeptide containing the complete amino acid sequence (DeJongh et al. 1991).

Messenger RNA transcribed from the second gene, Caα_1/2, appears in two alternatively spliced forms: Caα_1/2a mRNA codes for the α_1 subunit found in cardiac muscle, while Caα_1/2b mRNA is expressed in smooth muscle tissue (Biel et al. 1991). The major distinction between the translation products of these two forms is in the IVS3 segment, which differs as a result of the alternative splicing (Perez-Reyes et al. 1990). In addition, the two splice variants are differentially expressed during cardiac development (Diebold et al. 1992).

cDNAs representing a third gene, Caα_1/3, were isolated from endocrine cell (Seino et al. 1992) and neuronal tissue (Williams et al. 1992a) cDNA libraries. They represent a DHP-sensitive α_1 subunit.

Binding sites for organic compounds have been identified by photoaffinity labelling of skeletal muscle α_1 subunits with compounds of interest, followed by limited proteolysis and immunoprecipitation to isolate labelled peptides. By this approach, DHP binding sites were localized to the S5 to S6 loop region of domain III (Striessnig et al. 1991; Nakayama et al. 1991) and to a cytoplasmic portion of the molecule following segment IVS6 (Regulla et al. 1991). The PAA binding site was found to be immediately after transmembrane segment of IVS6 (Striessnig et al. 1990).

cDNAs representing the genes for DHP-*in*sensitive α_1 subunits have been isolated from neuronal tissues or from cell lines of neuronal origin. A major difference between the translated amino acid sequences of these cDNAs and those of DHP-*sensitive* α_1 subunits is the presence of a large hydrophilic intracellular segment between domains II and III of the DHP-insensitive α_1 subunits.

Caα_1/4, isolated from rat brain (Starr et al. 1991), shares 33% sequence identity with the α_1 subunits of cardiac and skeletal muscle. Caα_1/4 is expressed in all regions of the rat central nervous system, but most prominently in the cerebellum. Transient expression of Caα_1/4 RNA in frog oocytes results in high-voltage-activated Ca^{2+} currents that are insensitive to DHPs and ω-conotoxin, but are inhibited by ω-AgaIVA, thus characterizing this Caα_1/4 subunit as a P-type calcium channel (Mori et al. 1991).

Caα_1/5 mRNA has also been isolated from rat brain (Dubel et al. 1992) and is specifically expressed in neurons. The translation product of the Caα_1/5 gene is irreversibly blocked by ω-conotoxin, identifying this α_1 subunit as the N-type calcium channel (Williams et al. 1992b).

The RNA coding for another α_1 subunit, Caα_1/6, was isolated recently from rabbit brain (Niidome et al. 1992). The Caα_1/6 sequence is highly homologous to Caα_1/4 and Caα_1/5 sequences. Like Caα_1/5, Caα_1/6 is expressed in brain only, most prominently in the hippocampus. Pharmacological properties of Caα_1/6 have yet to be reported.

The β Subunit

The β subunits of voltage-sensitive calcium channels comprise a class of 60–70 kDa proteins which are phosphorylated by cAMP-dependent protein kinases, phosphokinase-C (PKC), and cGMP-dependent kinases (Curtis and Catterall 1985; Takahashi et al. 1987; Jahn et al. 1988). They are not glycosylated and do not copurify with membranes (Takahashi et al. 1987). Also, since analysis of their primary structure has revealed no putative membrane-spanning domains, β subunits are thought to interact with α_1 subunits on the intracellular side of the plasma membrane.

Studies of the coexpression of skeletal muscle β and α_1, subunits have shown that the β subunit has profound effects on the activation and inactivation kinetics of the α_1 subunit (Varadi et al. 1991; Lacerda et al. 1991). Furthermore, an increase in both the number of DHP binding sites (Varadi et al. 1991) and the amplitude of peak currents (Varadi et al. 1991; Mori et al. 1991) has been observed upon coexpression of α_1 and β subunits as compared to expression of α_1 subunits alone.

Molecular cloning of cDNAs for calcium channel β subunits has so far revealed three distinct β genes (CaB1–CaB3) as well as several splice variants. The CaB1 gene codes for the β subunit CaB1a of the skeletal muscle calcium channel (Ruth et al. 1989). As reported by Powers et al. (1992), this same gene gives rise to two additional alternatively spliced products: replacement of a skeletal muscle-specific exon by a smaller exon generates CaB1b mRNA, which is expressed in brain (Williams et al. 1992b); substitution of the C-terminal portion of the CaB1b coding sequence through a second splicing event leads to CaB1c mRNA, which encodes a second species of brain-specific β subunit (Pragnell et al. 1991).

The CaB2 and CaB3 gene products have an overall homology with CaB1 of 71% and 66%, respectively. Four different alternative splice products of CaB2 have been identified so far as being expressed in heart and brain (Hullin et al. 1992; Perez-Reyes et al. 1992). The CaB3 transcript is expressed predominantly in brain, and to a minor extent in aorta, trachea, and lung (Hullin et al. 1992).

The α_2/δ Subunit

The α_2 and δ components of the VOCC were first isolated as co-precipitates of immunoprecipitated rabbit skeletal muscle DHP receptors (Ellis et al. 1988). cDNA cloning subsequently revealed that the two subunits are the product of a single gene, being translated from one mRNA and then processed into two proteins of 935 amino acids (α_2) and 144 amino acids (δ) (De Jongh et al. 1990). Both proteins are highly glycosylated and bind neither DHP nor PAA (Ellis et al. 1988). Hydropathy analyses suggest that the δ

subunit has one transmembrane spanning segment with an intracellular C- and an extracellular N-terminus. The molecular structure of the α_2 subunit is not yet clear: some authors have described α_2 as an extracellular protein that is anchored in the membrane by the δ subunit (Jay et al. 1991; Hullin et al. 1993); others have defined two transmembrane segments for the α_2 subunit, with both N- and C-termini being extracellular (Catterall 1991).

The α_2/δ subunit is highly conserved in different tissues and among species. cDNA clones isolated from the RNAs of rabbit skeletal muscle (Ellis et al. 1988), human brain, and rat brain (Kim et al. 1992; Williams et al. 1992b) share more than 95% sequence homology. The skeletal muscle α_2 subunit and the α_2 subunit expressed predominantly in brain are alternative mRNA splicing variants differing at two sites: in comparison to the skeletal muscle α_2 subunit, the brain-specific translation product carries an insertion of 7 amino acids at the first site and a deletion of 19 amino acids at the second.

It has been reported that coexpression in oocytes of the cardiac α_1 subunit with α_2 and δ subunits from skeletal muscle enhances Ca^{2+} currents and fine-tunes activation kinetics as compared to expression of the α_1 subunit alone (Singer et al. 1991). Further, coexpression of skeletal muscle α_2/δ and β subunits with cardiac (Singer et al. 1991) and brain (Mori et al. 1991) α_1 subunits shows synergistic effects on the enhancement of calcium currents.

The γ Subunit

The γ subunit is the smallest subunit of the calcium channel complex (Campbell et al. 1988; Catterall et al. 1988). A cDNA clone having an open reading frame coding for a protein of 222 amino acids was isolated from rabbit skeletal muscle (Jay et al. 1990).

The molecular weight of the γ subunit, calculated from the cDNA sequence, is 25 kDa. This agrees with data obtained from SDS-PAGE analysis of immunoprecipitated VOCC protein, which showed apparent molecular weights of 32 kDa for the glycosylated γ subunit (Campbell et al. 1988; Catterall et al. 1988), and 20 kDa for its nonglycosylated form (Takahashi et al. 1987).

RNA expression studies have revealed that the γ subunit is present only in skeletal muscle. Other tissues that have been examined, such as cardiac muscle, brain, liver, and kidney, showed no expression of γ subunit mRNA (Jay et al. 1990).

Biochemical studies (Campbell et al. 1988; Catterall et al. 1988) and computer analysis predict a structure with four transmembrane-spanning segments and intracellular N- and C-termini (Jay et al. 1990). Biochemical data have indicated that the γ subunit has two extracellular N-linked glycosylation sites, and computer analysis showed two potential phosphorylation sites in the intracellular portion of the γ subunit (Jay et al. 1990).

There has been one report that the γ subunit accelerates inactivation processes and enhances the voltage sensitivity of the channel when coexpressed with cardiac α_1 in oocytes (Singer et al. 1991).

Regulation of Voltage-Dependent Calcium Channel Activation

Activation of voltage-operated calcium channels by changes in the membrane potential is modulated by a variety of hormones and transmitters (Hess 1990). Although there is general agreement that GTP-binding proteins are involved in signal transduction, the exact mechanism of coupling between G-proteins and the VOCC is still under dispute.

Transmitter-mediated down-regulation of calcium channel activity has been reported to be dependent on PKC in neuronal cells of dorsal root ganglia (Rane and Dunlap 1986), whereas the interaction between transmitter receptors and calcium channels in other neuronal cells seems to be independent of PKC (Wanke et al. 1987).

Two contradictory sets of data attribute the positive inotropic effect of beta-adrenergic stimulation on the heart muscle on the one hand to a PKA-mediated phosphorylation of the cardiac calcium channel (Hartzell et al. 1991; Hartzell and Fischmeister 1992), or on the other to a direct interaction between the channel and G-proteins (Yatani and Brown 1989). Recent evidence suggests that cAMP-dependent phosphorylation of cardiac and vascular calcium channels may be dependent on the presence of the β subunit (Klöckner et al. 1992). Thus, the mechanism of beta-adrenergic stimulation may also depend on the subunit composition of calcium channel complexes (Hullin et al. 1993).

Apart from the interaction between calcium channels and hormone or transmitter receptors, feedback regulation of calcium channel activity via phosphorylation of the channel by Ca^{2+}/calmodulin-dependent protein kinase II has been described for smooth muscle (McCarron et al. 1992) as well as for calcium channels of other tissues (Tsien and Tsien 1990).

Summary

The central role of voltage-operated calcium channels in regulating Ca^{2+} homeostasis in excitable cells has made these channels important sites for pharmacological intervention. The development of subtype-specific channel ligands has become a high priority in drug discovery programs aimed at the modulation of human neuronal Ca^{2+} channels. At the same time, the ubiquity of calcium channels, and their similarity in different tissues, has made difficult the identification of agents with specific pharmacologic effects on VOCCs of only one or another cell type.

However, the diversity of calcium channels that has been uncovered in recent molecular biological studies of the microheterogeneity of channel subunits has encouraged the development of in vitro drug screening systems that would greatly facilitate the discovery of highly selective calcium channel antagonists and agonists. The messenger RNAs coding for different tissue- or developmental stage-specific subtypes of calcium channel subunits have been cloned, and single functional channel types can be displayed abundantly on the surface of stably transfected mammalian host cells. Such recombinantly expressed Ca^{2+} channel genes provide a unique opportunity for the rapid identification and pharmacological characterization of novel ligands of voltage operated Ca^{2+} channels.

In the near future, the availability of cloned and expressed Ca^{2+} channels will allow critical assessment of the various drug binding sites at the molecular level, ultimately providing a rational course of pharmacological optimization of newly discovered Ca^{2+} channel ligands.

References

Bean BP (1989) Classes of calcium channels in vertebrate cells. Annu Rev Physiol 51:367–384

Biel M, Ruth P, Bosse E, Hullin R, Stühmer W, Flockerzi V, Hofmann F (1990) Primary structure and functional expression of a high voltage activated calcium channel from rabbit lung. FEBS Lett 269:409–412

Biel M, Hullin R, Freundner S, Singer D, Dascal N, Flockerzi V, Hofmann F (1991) Tissue-specific expression of high-voltage-activated dihydropyridine-sensitive L-type calcium channels. Eur J Biochem 200:81–88

Campbell KP, Leung AT, Sharp AH (1988) The biochemistry and molecular biology of the dihydropyridine-sensitive calcium channel. Trends Neurosci 11:425–430

Catterall WA (1991) Functional subunit structure of voltage-gated calcium channels. Science 253:1499–1500

Catterall WA, Striessnig J (1992) Receptor sites for Ca^{2+}-channel antagonists. Trends Pharmacol Sci 13:256–262

Catterall WA, Seagar MJ, Takahashi M (1988) Molecular properties of dihydropyridine-sensitive calcium channels in skeletal muscle. J Biol Chem 263:3535–3538

Cruz LJ, Olivera BM (1986) Calcium channel antagonists. Omega-conotoxin defines a new high affinity site. J Biol Chem 261:6230–6233

Curtis BM, Catterall WA (1985) Phosphorylation of the calcium antagonist receptor of the voltage-sensitive calcium channel by cAMP-dependent protein kinase. Proc Natl Acad Sci USA 82:2528–2532

De Jongh KS, Warner C, Catterall WA (1990) Subunits of purified calcium channels: α_2 and δ are encoded by the same gene. J Biol Chem 265:14738–14741

De Jongh KS, Warner C, Colvin AA, Catterall WA (1991) Characterization of the two size forms of the α_1 subunit of skeletal muscle L-type calcium channels. Proc Natl Acad Sci USA 88:10778–10782

Diebold RJ, Koch WJ, Ellinor PT, Wang J-J, Muthuchamy M, Wieczorek DF, Schwartz A (1992) Mutually exclusive exon splicing of the cardiac calcium channel α_1 subunit gene generates developmentally regulated isoforms in the rat heart. Proc Natl Acad Sci USA 89:1497–1501

Dubel SJ, Starr TV, Hell J, Ahlijanian MK, Enyeart J, Catterall WA, Snutch TP (1992) Molecular cloning of the α_1 subunit of an ω-conotoxin-sensitive calcium channel. Proc Natl Acad Sci USA 89:5058–5062

Ellis SB, Williams ME, Ways NR, Brenner R, Sharp AH, Leung AT, Campbell KP, McKenna E, Koch WJ, Hui A, Schwartz A, Harpold MM (1988) Sequence and expression of mRNAs encoding the α_1 and α_2 subunits of a DHP-sensitive calcium channel. Science 241:1661–1664

Grabner M, Friedrich K, Knaus H-G, Striessnig J, Scheffauer F, Staudinger R, Koch WJ, Schwartz A, Glossmann H (1991) Calcium channels from *Cyprinus carpio* skeletal muscle. Proc Natl Acad Sci USA 88:727–731

Guy HR, Conti F (1990) Pursuing the structure and function of voltage-gated channels. Trends Neurol Sci 13:201–206

Hartzell HC, Fischmeister R (1992) Direct regulation of cardiac calcium channels by G-proteins: neither proven nor needed? Trends Pharmacol Sci 13:380–385

Hartzell HC, Mery P-F, Fischmeister R, Szabo G (1991) Sympathetic regulation of cardiac calcium current is due exclusively to cAMP-dependent phosphorylation. Nature 351:573–576

Heinemann SH, Terlau H, Stühmer W, Imoto K, Numa S (1992) Calcium channel characteristics conferred on the sodium channel by single mutations. Nature 356:441–443

Hess P (1990) Calcium channels in vertebrate cells. Annu Rev Neurosci 13:337–356

Hui AS, Ellinor PT, Wang J, Schwartz A (1991) Molecular cloning of multiple subtypes of a novel rat brain isoform of the α_1 subunit of the voltage-dependent calcium channel. Neuron 7:35–41

Hullin R, Singer-Lahat D, Freichel M, Biel M, Dascal N, Hofmann F, Flockerzi V (1992) Calcium channel β-subunit heterogeneity: functional expression of cloned cDNA from heart, aorta and brain. EMBO J 11:885–890

Hullin R, Biel M, Flockerzi V, Hofmann F (1993) Tissue-specific expression of calcium channels. Trends Cardiovasc Med 3:48–53

Jahn H, Nastainczyk W, Röhrkasten A, Schneider T, Hofmann F (1988) Site-specific phosphorylation of the purified receptor for calcium-channel blockers by cAMP- and cGMP-dependent protein kinases, protein kinase C, calmodulin-dependent protein kinase II and casein kinase II. Eur J Biochem 178:535–542

Jay DS, Ellis SB, McCue AF, Williams ME, Vedvick TS, Harpold MM, Campbell KP (1990) Primary structure of the γ subunit of the DHP-sensitive calcium channel from skeletal muscle. Science 248:490–492

Jay DS, Sharp AH, Kahl SD, Vedvick TS, Harpold MM, Campbell KP (1991) Structural characterization of the dihydropyridine-sensitive calcium channel α_2-subunit and the associated δ peptides. J Biol Chem 266:3287–3293

Kamb A, Iverson LE, Tanouye MA (1987) Molecular characterization of Shaker, a *Drosophila* gene, that encodes a potassium channel. Cell 50:405–413

Kennedy MB (1989) Regulation of neuronal function by calcium. Trends Neurosci 12:417–420

Kim H-L, Kim H, Lee P, King RG, Chin H (1992) Rat brain expresses an alternatively spliced form of the dihydropyridine-sensitive L-type calcium channel α_2 subunit. Proc Natl Acad Sci USA 89:3251–3255

Klöckner U, Itagaki K, Bodi I, Schwartz A (1992) β-subunit expression is required for cAMP-dependent increase of cloned cardiac and vascular calcium channel currents. Pflügers Arch 420:413–415

Koch WJ, Ellinor PT, Schwartz A (1990) cDNA cloning of a DHP-sensitive calcium channel from rat aorta. J Biol Chem 265:17786–17791

Lacerda AE, Kim HS, Ruth P, Perez-Reyes E, Flockerzi V, Hofmann F, Birnbaumer L, Brown AM (1991) Normalization of current kinetics by interaction between the α_1 and β subunits of the skeletal muscle dihydropyridine-sensitive Ca^{2+} channel. Nature 352:527–530

Marty A (1989) The physiological role of calcium-dependent channels. Trends Neurosci 12:420–424

McCarron JG, McGeown JG, Reardon S, Ikebe M, Fay FS, Walsh JV (1992) Calcium-dependent enhancement of calcium current in smooth muscle by calmodulin-dependent protein kinase II. Nature 357:74–77

Mikami A, Imoto K, Tanabe T, Niidome T, Mori Y, Takeshima H, Narumiya S, Numa S (1989) Primary structure and functional expression of the cardiac dihydropyridine-sensitive calcium channel. Nature 340:230–233

Mintz IM, Venema VJ, Swiderek K, Lee T, Bean BP, Adams ME (1992) P-type calcium channels blocked by the spider toxin ω-Aga-IVA. Nature 355:827–829

Morgan JI, Curran T (1989) Stimulus-transcription coupling in neurons: role of cellular immediate-early genes. Trends Neurosci 12:459–462

Mori Y, Friedrich T, Kim M-S, Mikami A, Nakai J, Ruth P, Bosse E, Hofmann F, Flockerzi V, Furuichi F, Mikoshiba K, Imoto K, Tanabe T, Numa S (1991) Primary structure and functional expression from complementary DNA of a brain calcium channel. Nature 350:398–402

Nakayama H, Taki M, Striessnig J, Glossmann H, Catterall WA, Kanaoka Y (1991) Identification of 1,4-dihydropyridine binding regions within the α_1 subunit of skeletal muscle Ca^{2+}-channels by photoaffinity labeling with diazipine. Proc Natl Acad Sci USA 88:9203–9207

Niidome T, Kim M-S, Friedrich T, Mori Y (1992) Molecular cloning and characterization of a novel calcium channel from rabbit brain. FEBS Lett 308:7–13

Noda M, Shimizu S, Tanabe H, Takai T, Kayamo T, Ikeda T, Takahashi H, Nakayama H, Knaoka Y, Minamino N, Kangawa K, Matsuo H, Raftery MA, Hirose T, Inagama S, Hayashida H, Miyata T, Numa S (1984) Primary structure of *Electrophorus electricus* sodium channel deduced from cDNA sequence. Nature 312:121–127

Perez-Reyes E, Wei X, Castellano A, Birnbaumer L (1990) Molecular diversity of L-type calcium channels. J Biol Chem 265:20430–20436

Perez-Reyes E, Castellano A, Kim HS, Bertrand P, Baggstrom E, Lacerda AE, Wei X, Birnbaumer L (1992) Cloning and expression of a cardiac/brain β-subunit of the L-type calcium channel. J Biol Chem 267:1792–1797

Powers PA, Liu S, Hogan K, Gregg RG (1992) Skeletal muscle and brain isoforms of a β-subunit of human voltage-dependent calcium channels are encoded by a single gene. J Biol Chem 267:22967–22972

Pragnell M, Sakamoto J, Jay SD, Campbell KP (1991) Cloning and tissue-specific expression of the brain calcium channel β-subunit. FEBS Lett 291:253–258

Rane SG, Dunlap K (1986) Kinase C activator 1,2-oleoylacetylglycerol attenuates voltage dependent calcium current in sensory neurons. Proc Natl Acad Sci USA 83:184–188

Regulla S, Schneider T, Nastainczyk W, Meyer HE, Hofmann F (1991) Identification of the site of interaction of the dihydropyridine channel blockers nitrendipine and azidopine with the calcium channel α_1 subunit. EMBO J 10:45–49
Ruth P, Röhrkasten A, Biel M, Bosse E, Regulla S, Meyer HE, Flockerzi V, Hofmann F (1989) Primary structure of the β subunit of the DHP-sensitive calcium channel from skeletal muscle. Science 245:1115–1118
Seino S, Chen L, Seino M, Blondel O, Takeda J, Johnson JH, Bell GI (1992) Cloning of the α_1 subunit of a voltage-dependent calcium channel expressed in pancreatic β cells. Proc Natl Acad Sci USA 89:584–588
Sheng M, Greenberg ME (1990) The regulation and function of c-fos and other immediate early genes in the nervous system. Neuron 4:477–485
Singer D, Biel M, Lotan I, Flockerzi V, Hofmann F, Dascol N (1991) The role of the subunits in the function of the calcium channel. Science 253:1553–1556
Snutch TP, Leonard JP, Gilbert MM, Lester IA, Davidson N (1990) Rat brain expresses a heterogeneous family of calcium channels. Proc Natl Acad Sci USA 87:3391–3395
Snutch TP, Tomlinson WJ, Leonard JP, Gilbert MM (1991) Distinct calcium channels are generated by alternative splicing and are differentially expressed in the mammalian CNS. Neuron 7:45–57
Soldatov NM (1992) Molecular diversity of L-type Ca^{2+}-channel transcripts in human fibroblasts. Proc Natl Acad Sci USA 89:4628–4632
Starr TV, Prystay W, Snutch TP (1991) Primary structure of a calcium channel that is highly expressed in the rat cerebellum. Proc Natl Acad Sci USA 88:5621–5625
Striessnig J, Glossmann H, Catterall WA (1990) Identification of a phenylalkylamine binding region within the α_1 subunit of skeletal muscle Ca^{2+}-channels. Proc Natl Acad Sci USA 87:9108–9112
Striessnig J, Murphy BJ, Catterall WA (1991) Dihydropyridine receptor of L-type Ca^{2+}-channels: identification of binding domains for (^{3}H) (+)-PN200-110 and (^{3}H) azidopine within the α_1 subunit. Proc Natl Acad Sci USA 88:10769–10773
Stühmer W, Conti F, Suzuki H, Wang X, Noda M, Yahagi N, Kubo H, Numa S (1989) Structural parts involved in activation and inactivation of the sodium channel. Nature 339:597–603
Takahashi M, Seagar MJ, Jones JF, Reber BFX, Catterall WA (1987) Subunit structure of dihydropyridine-sensitive calcium channels from skeletal muscle. Proc Natl Acad Sci USA 84:5478–5482
Tanabe T, Takeshima H, Mikami A, Flockerzi V, Takahashi H, Kangawa K, Kojima M, Matsuo H, Hirose T, Numa S (1987) Primary structure of the receptor for calcium channel blockers from skeletal muscle. Nature 328:313–318
Tsien RW (1983) Calcium channels in excitable cell membranes. Annu Rev Physiol 45:341–358
Tsien RW, Tsien RY (1990) Calcium channels, stores and oscillations. Annu Rev Cell Biol 6:715–760
Tsien RW, Ellinor PT, Horne WA (1991) Molecular diversity of voltage-dependent Ca^{2+} channels. Trends Pharmacol Sci 12:349–354
Varadi G, Lory P, Schultz D, Varadi M, Schwartz A (1991) Acceleration of activation and inactivation by the β subunit of the skeletal muscle calcium channel. Nature 352:159–162

Wanke E, Ferroni A, Malgaroli A, Ambrosini A, Pozzan T, Meldoseli J (1987) Activation of a muscarinic receptor selectively inhibits a rapidly inactivated calcium current in rat sympathetic neurons. Proc Natl Acad Sci USA 84:4314–4317

Williams ME, Brust PF, Feldman DH, Saraswathi P, Simerson S, Maroufi A, McCue AF, Velicelebi G, Ellis SB, Harpold MM (1992a) Structure and functional expression of an ω-conotoxin-sensitive human N-type calcium channel. Science 257:389–394

Williams ME, Feldmann DH, McCue AF, Brenner R, Velicelebi G, Ellis SB, Harpold MM (1992b) Structure and functional expression of α_1, α_2, and β subunits of a novel human neuronal calcium channel subtype. Neuron 8:71–84

Yatani Y, Brown AM (1989) Rapid β-adrenergic modulation of cardiac calcium channel currents by a fast G-protein pathway. Science 245:71–74

From the Cardiovascular to the Central Nervous System – An Adventure in the Pharmacology of Dihydropyridines

A. Scriabine

My interest in Ca^{2+} antagonists dates back to the early 1970s. After having read the initial publications of Fleckenstein [1,2], I suggested to the management of a pharmaceutical company, which employed me at that time, a research project involving a search for novel Ca^{2+} antagonists. In the opinion of the research management, however, the blockade of Ca^{2+} entry into the cells was most likely to be associated with severe side effects, so that Ca^{2+} antagonists were not likely to succeed. The company entered the Ca^{2+} antagonist field eventually with a licensed "me-too" compound, but 10–15 years too late.

Even though I anticipated the usefulness of Ca^{2+} antagonists in the treatment of angina pectoris and hypertension, I never visualized how large the potential market for Ca^{2+} antagonists was likely to be. As Fig. 1 indicates, it exceeded 2 billion dollars in 1991 in the USA alone. This number refers almost exclusively to their use in the treatment of cardiovascular diseases. The only noncardiovascular indication approved in the USA is that for nimodipine, in the prevention of neurological deficits associated with subarachnoid hemorrhage. Since the list of current or potential indications for Ca^{2+} antagonists is continuously expanding (Table 1), the market size is likely to double during the next 3–5 years.

The pioneering work of Bayer scientists in the field of Ca^{2+} antagonists was one of the reasons I joined Miles. I had heard about a pipeline full of new dihydropyridines which were selective for either the coronary, peripheral, or cerebral vasculature, and I was anxious to participate in their development. Subsequently, the selectivity of nimodipine for the cerebral circulation was confirmed, while the selectivity of other dihydropyridines for either peripheral or coronary vascular beds remained questionable, particularly under clinical conditions. Nevertheless, the second generation Ca^{2+} antagonists, nitrendipine and nisoldipine, had more favorable vasodilator/cardiac depressant activity ratios than either verapamil or nifedipine and had a longer duration of action [3,4]. At Miles we were able to correlate their ability to inhibit $^{45}Ca^{2+}$ uptake into vascular tissue with their vasodilator action, to demonstrate differences in their receptor binding properties,

Miles Institute for Preclinical Pharmacology, West Haven, CT 06516, USA

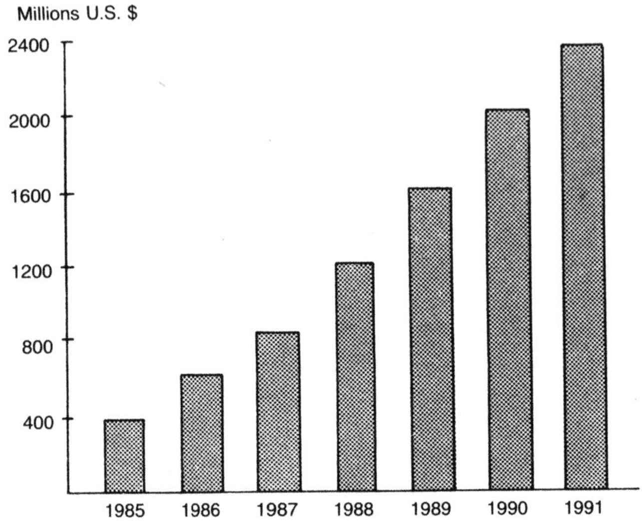

Fig. 1. Ca^{2+} antagonist market in the USA

and to differentiate some of their vascular effects from those of verapamil [5–7].

In addition to experimental studies performed at the Miles Institute for Preclinical Pharmacology in New Haven, we supported extramural studies with Bayer Ca^{2+} antagonists in many North American academic laboratories. Some of these studies led to the demonstration of certain advantages of either nitrendipine or nisoldipine in comparison to nifedipine and to other Ca^{2+} channel antagonists. Nitrendipine, for example, was shown to have a superior therapeutic index (ratio of coronary vasodilator to cardiac depressant effects) than either nifedipine, verapamil, or diltiazem [8] and to protect kidneys or liver from ischemic damage [9,10]. The selectivity of nimodipine for cerebral circulation was confirmed by Haws and Heistad in rabbits [11], while McCalden et al. demonstrated a cerebral vasodilator effect of this drug at very low doses in baboons [12].

We suspected that the beneficial effects of nimodipine in the prevention of neurological deficits following subarachnoid hemorrhage [13] could not be explained solely by its cerebral vasodilator activity, and we initiated electrophysiological studies with this drug at Miles and in academic laboratories. The studies led to the discovery by McCarthy that nimodipine, at low nanomolar concentrations, blocks Ca^{2+} currents through L-type Ca^{2+} channels in mammalian neurones [14]. After the introduction of Ca^{2+} imaging technology at the Miles Institute for Preclinical Pharmacology, Chisholm et al. [15,16] demonstrated that nimodipine antagonizes K^+-induced elevation of free cytosolic Ca^{2+} in isolated rat hippocampal neurones (Fig. 2). A possible relationship between these effects of nimodipine and its

Table 1. Current and potential indications for Ca^{2+} antagonists

Cardiovascular	
Hypertension[a]	Atherosclerosis[a]
Coronary heart disease	Traumatic shock[a]
Cardioplegia	Congestive heart failure
Hypertrophic subaortic stenosis	Thrombosis
Peripheral vascular disease	Renal failure[a]
Arrhythmias	
Central nervous system	
Subarachnoid hemorrhage	Dementia
Cerebral Ischemia[a]	Alzheimer's
Global	Vascular
Focal	Multi-infarct
Migraine	Head trauma
Age-associated memory dysfunction[a]	Spinal cord trauma[a]
Alcholism[a]	Depression
Preference	Learning deficits[a]
Withdrawal	Hearing disorders
Intoxication	Survival of brain transplants[a]
Cocaine intoxication[a]	Parkinson's Disease
Amphetamine abuse[a]	Spinal cord injury
Opiate withdrawal	Prevention of brain damage during delivery[a]
Retraction-induced brain damage[a]	
Respiratory system	
Pulmonary hypertension[a]	
Asthma	
Esophageal achalasia	
Gynecological and obstetrical	
Primary dysmenorrhea	
Premature labor[a]	
Cancer chemotherapy	
Prevention of cancer cell resistance to anticancer drugs	
Prevention of metastases[a]	
Prevention of cardiotoxicity of doxorubicin	
Prevention of neurotoxicity of cisplatin	

[a] Indications supported by North American studies.

potential usefulness in the therapy of Alzheimer's disease was suggested by the more recent findings of Chisholm et al. [17], that β-amyloid fragment [25–35] increases cytoplasmic free Ca^{2+} in hippocampal cells and that nimodipine, at low nanomolar concentrations, antagonizes this effect (Fig. 3).

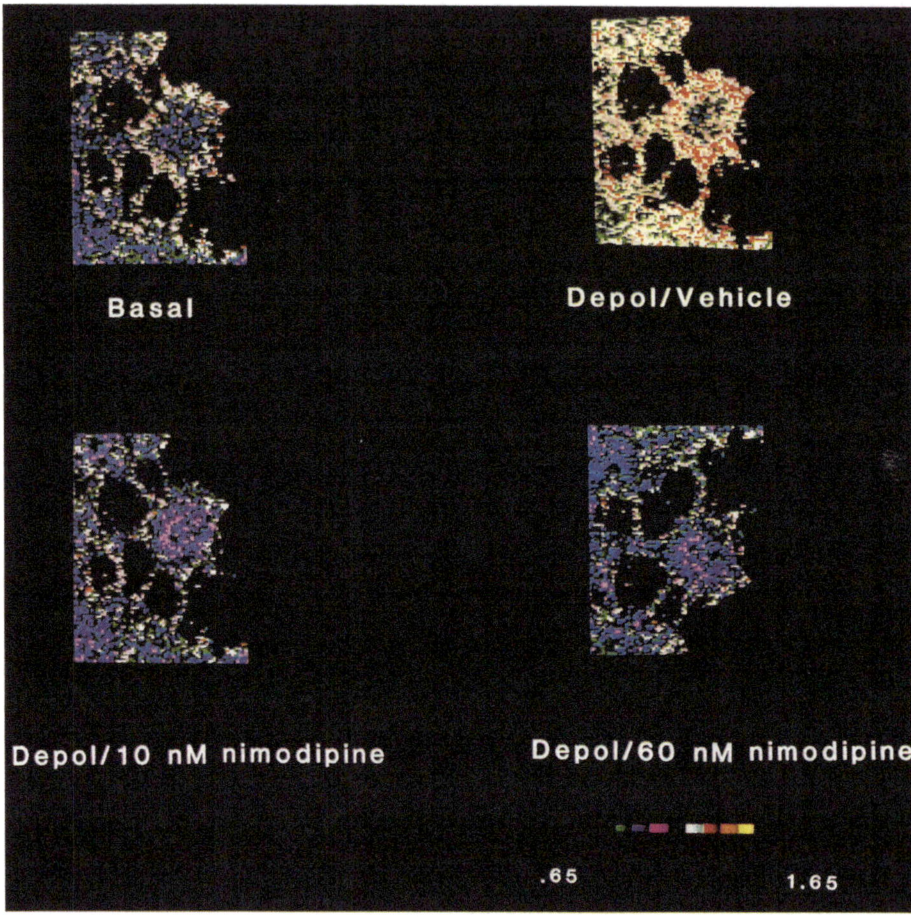

Fig. 2. Digitized image of the $[Ca^{2+}]_i$-dependent fura-2 ratio obtained from a single neuron under basal conditions (1 m*M* $[K^+]_e$) (*upper left*), during depolarization (55 m*M* $[K^+]_e$) in the presence of vehicle (PEG 400) (*upper right*), 10 n*M* (*lower left*), and 60 n*M* nimodipine (*lower right*) applied during continued depolarization. Pseudocolor scale is linear with ratio (340 nm/380 nm). Here, 0.65–1.65 represents 150–350 n*M* Ca^{2+}. (From [16])

The effects of nimodipine on the central nervous system were also studied extensively at various North American academic institutions. These studies provided additional experimental evidence for the neuroprotective action of nimodipine. Nimodipine was proposed to inhibit neuronal Ca^{2+} overload caused by ischemia-induced depolarization of the cell membrane. This mechanism was accepted by most investigators as a working hypothesis, although some investigators failed to confirm neuroprotection or attributed it to other activities of the drug, e.g., free radical scavenging. The highlights

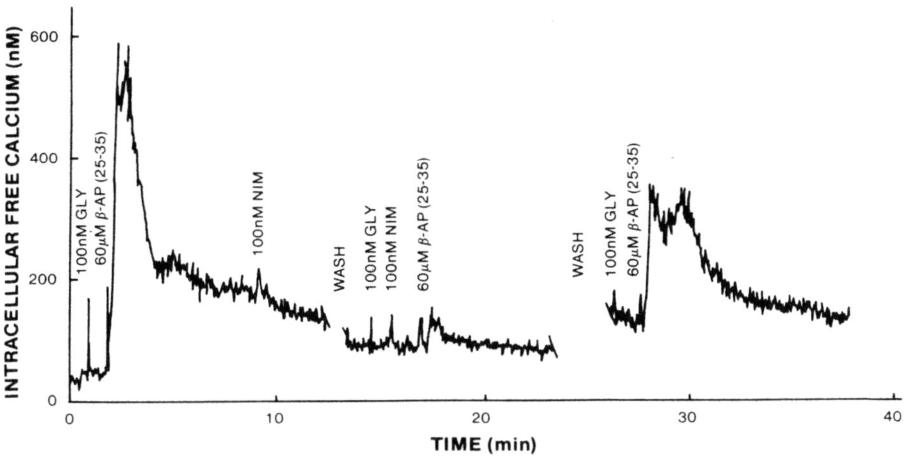

Fig. 3. Nimodipine block of $[Ca^{2+}]_i$ responses to a toxic amyloid fragment, β-AP [25–35], in a rat hippocampal neuron. $[Ca^{2+}]_i$ was measured using ratiometric fura-2 methods. Nimodipine or amyloid fragment were applied where indicated and were present until washout. The same neuron was challenged with β-AP three times. In the presence of nimodipine (*NIM*) the amyloid fragment had no effect on $[Ca^{2+}]_i$. This experiment was repeated eight times with similar results. (Courtesy of J. Chisholm)

of this program included: demonstration of the beneficial effects of nimodipine on neurological deficits caused by transient cerebral ischemia in pig-tailed monkeys [18], reduction of neurological scores in baboons subjected to middle cerebral artery occlusion [19], and cognition enhancement in aging rats, rabbits, and monkeys [20–22]. Strong support in favor of the involvement of cytoplasmic free Ca^{2+} in the neuroprotective action of nimodipine was provided by Uematsu et al. [23], who demonstrated that, by intravenous infusion to cats subjected to the occlusion of middle cerebral arteries, nimodipine prevents the rise of free cytosolic Ca^{2+} and reduces histologic brain damage.

In cell cultures nimodipine antagonized various neurotoxins. In mixed cortical cell cultures, containing both neuronal and glial elements, nimodipine at micromolar concentrations reduced α-amino-3-hydroxy-5-methyl-4-isoxazolepropionic acid (AMPA)- or kainate-induced neurotoxicity [24]. Elevation of Ca^{2+} in hippocampal neurones by the HIV envelope protein gp120 was found to be reduced by nimodipine [25]. In addition to its neuronal effects, nimodipine was found to control Ca^{2+} entry into glial cells as well. Depolarization-induced Ca^{2+} elevation in astrocytes was reduced by nimodipine at low nanomolar range [26].

The relevance of the in vitro demonstrated neuroprotective action of nimodipine to the in vivo situation was supported by studies in lesioned animals. Nimodipine was reported to protect cells in the medial septal region after unilateral surgical destruction of the fornix [27]. At 15 mg/kg po nimodipine enhanced recovery of higher cognitive or sensorimotor-integrative tasks after acute, focal brain lesions in the rat [28]. In the eight-arm radial maze studies nimodipine enhanced the retention of learned tasks of rats with hippocampal lesions [29].

Of considerable potential interest for neurosurgeons was the demonstration by Zhou et al. [30] that nimodipine enhances survival of suboptimal neural grafts, possibly due to its angiogenic activity. This observation was recently extended by Horner and Stokes [31] to intraspinal fetal grafts in rats; their findings suggested the potential usefulness of the drug in spinal cord transplantation to improve survival of grafts and behavioral outcome.

Intensive studies with nimodipine in North America led to the discovery of numerous new indications and to the confirmation of some of the indications suggested by European investigators (Table 1). The studies also led to the realization of the limitations of nimodipine: limited bioavailability, relatively short duration of action and the fact that, in order to protect neuronal tissue from ischemic damage, nimodipine has to be administered as soon as possible after the insult and not 6 or 12 h later. Nimodipine can be expected to have the best effect in indications requiring preventive therapy. Time release formulations or novel delivery systems will have to be developed to assure the commercial success of the drug.

Summary

The second generation cardiovascular Ca^{2+} antagonists nitrendipine and nisoldipine were studied extensively in North America. Their relative selectivity for vascular smooth muscle as compared to myocardium was confirmed while their selectivity for coronary vs peripheral blood vessels remained questionable. Certain advantages of second generation Ca^{2+}-antagonists, e.g., superior therapeutic index and longer duration of action, were described.

The neuroprotective effect of nimodipine was demonstrated in vitro and in vivo. The effect was attributed to nimodipine-induced inhibition of Ca^{2+} currents through L-type channels. The same mechanism is thought to be responsible for nimodipine-induced cognition activation and learning enhancement in lesioned or aging rats. New clinical indications are likely to further expand the market for Ca^{2+} antagonists.

References

1. Fleckenstein A, Tritthart H, Fleckenstein B, Herbst A, Grün G (1969) Eine neue Gruppe kompetitiver Ca^{2+} Antagonisten (iproveratril, D-600, prenylamine) mit starken Hemmeffekten auf die elektromechanische Koppelung im Warmblütermyokard. Pflugers Arch 359:R51

2. Fleckenstein A (1977) Specific pharmacology of calcium in myocardium, cardiac pacemakers and vascular smooth muscle. Annu Rev Pharmacol Toxicol 17:149–166
3. Stoepel K, Heise A, Kazda S (1981) Pharmacological studies of the antihypertensive effect of nitrendipine. Arzneimittelforschung 31:2056–2061
4. Kazda S, Garthoff B, Meyer H, Schloßmann K, Stoepel K, Towart R, Vater W, Wehinger E (1980) Pharmacology of a new calcium antagonistic compound, isobutyl methyl 1,4-dihydro-2,6-dimethyl-4-(2-nitrophenyl)-3, 5-pyridinedicarboxylate (nisoldipine, BAY K 5552). Arzneimittelforschung 30:2144–2162
5. Scriabine A, Johnson CE, Anderson CL, Steinsland OS, Janis RA (1984) Ca^{2+} channel inhibitory effects of nitrendipine on isolated rabbit arteries. In: Scriabine A, Vanov S, Deck K (eds) Nitrendipine. Urban and Schwarzenberg, Baltimore, pp 281–292
6. Scriabine A, Janis RA (1990) Recent developments in the pharmacology of Ca^{2+} antagonists. In: Yamada K, Shibata S (eds) Recent advances in calcium channels and calcium antagonists. Pergamon, New York, pp 77–84
7. Steinsland OS, Johnson CE, Scriabine A (1985) Comparative effects of nitrendipine and verapamil on neuroeffector transmission in the rabbit ear artery. J Cardiovasc Pharmacol 7:990–995
8. Lathrop DA, DiSalvo J, Dube GP, Schwartz A (1984) Electromechanical effects of calcium channel inhibitors in isolated canine Purkinje strands and potassium contracted coronary vascular smooth muscle. In: Scriabine A, Vanov S, Deck K (eds) Nitrendipine. Urban and Schwarzenberg, Baltimore, pp 185–198
9. Scriabine A, Anderson CL, Janis RA, Kojima K, Rasmussen H, Lee S, Michal U (1984) Some recent pharmacological findings with nitrendipine. J Cardiovasc Pharmacol 6:S937–S943
10. Thurman RG, Apel E, Lemasters JJ (1988) Protection of liver by calcium entry blockers. J Cardiovasc Pharmacol 12 (S4):S113–S116
11. Haws CW, Gourley JK, Heistad DD (1983) Effects of nimodipine on cerebral blood flow. J Pharmacol Exp Ther 225:24–28
12. McCalden TA, Nath RG, Thiele K (1984) The effect of a calcium antagonist (nimodipine) on basal cerebral blood flow and reactivity to various agonists. Stroke 15:527–530
13. Pickard JD, Murray GD, Illingworth R, Shaw MDM, Teasdale GM, Foy PM, Humphrey PRD, Lang DA, Nelson R, Richards P, Sinar J, Bailey S, Skene A (1989) Effect of oral nimodipine on cerebral infarction and outcome after subarachnoid hemorrhage: British Aneurism Nimodipine Trial. Br Med J 298:636–642
14. McCarthy RT (1989) Nimodipine block of L-type calcium channels in dorsal root ganglion cells. In: Traber J, Gispen WH (eds) Nimodipine and central nervous system function: new vistas: proceedings of the international workshop. Schattauer, Stuttgart, pp 35–49
15. Chisholm JC, Hunnicut EJ, Davis JN (1991) Potent nimodipine inhibition of elevated intracellular Ca^{2+} in depolarized hippocampal neurons, abstract S22. Special Poster Session 31st Annu Am Soc Cell Biol
16. Chisholm JC, Hunnicut EJ, Davis JN (1993) Neuronal Ca^{2+} responses to different classes of calcium lowering agents. Drugs in Development 2:117–126
17. Chisholm JC, Davis JN, Hunnicut EJ Jr (1992) Nimodipine-sensitive, β-amyloid (25–35)-induced $[Ca^{2+}]_i$ responses in single cultured rat hippocampal neurons. Abs Soc Neurosci 18:1439

18. Steen PA, Gisvold SE, Milde JH, Newberg LA, Scheithauer BW, Lanier WL, Michenfelder JD (1985) Nimodipine improves outcome when given after complete cerebral ischemia in primates. Anesthesiology 62:406–414
19. Hadley MN, Zabramski JM, Spetzler RF, Rigamonti D, Fifield MS (1989) The efficacy of intravenous nimodipine in the treatment of focal ischemia in a primate model. Neurosurgery 25:63–70
20. LeVere TE, Walker A (1991) Old age and cognition: enhancement of recent memory in aged rats by the calcium channel blocker nimodipine. Neurobiol Aging 13:63–66
21. Deyo RA, Straube KT, Disterhoft JF (1989) Nimodipine facilitates trace conditioning of the eye-blink response in aging rabbits. Science 243:809–811
22. Sandin M, Jasmin S, LeVere TE (1990) Aging and cognition: facilitation of recent memory in aged nonhuman primates by nimodipine. Neurobiol Aging 11:573–575
23. Uematsu D, Greenberg JH, Hickey WF, Reivich M (1989) Nimodipine attenuates both increase in cytosolic calcium and histologic damage following focal cerebral ischemia and reperfusion in cats. Stroke 20:1531–1537
24. Weiss JH, Choi DW (1991) Dihydropyridines attenuate slow excitatory amino acid neurotoxicity. In: Scriabine A, Teasdale GM, Tettenborn D, Young W (eds) Nimodipine. Pharmacological and clinical results in cerebral ischemia. Springer, Berlin Heidelberg New York, pp 57–63
25. Dreyer EB, Kaiser PK, Offerman JT, Lipton SA (1990) HIV-1 coat protein neurotoxicity prevented by calcium channel antagonists. Science 248:364–366
26. Hertz L, Bender AS, Woodbury DM, White HS (1989) Potassium-stimulated calcium uptake in astrocytes and its potent inhibition by nimodipine. J Neurosci Res 22:209–215
27. Isaacson RL, Shen Y, Mandel A (1990) Effects of nimodipine on medial septal area cells after section of the fimbria-fornix. Restor Neurol Neurosci 2:1–7
28. Anderson B, Finger S, Andersen CS, Hoagland N (1990) Sensorimotor cortical lesion effects and treatment with nimodipine. Physiol Behav 47:1045–1052
29. Finger S, Green L, Tarnoff ME, Mortman KD, Andersen A (1990) Nimodipine enhances learning after hippocampal damage. Exp Neurol 109:279–285
30. Zhou FC, Pu C-F, Finger S (1991) Nimodipne-enhanced survival of suboptimal neural grafts. Rest Neurol Neurosci 3:211–215
31. Horner PJ, Stokes BT (1992) Nimodipine enhances vascularity of intraspinal grafts and alters injury induced behavioral outcomes. Abs Soc Neurosci 18:1480

At the End of this Workshop . . .

Final Remarks

B. Garthoff

In a recent article in "Current Comments" (by Eugene Garfield in *Current Contents*, Jan. 18, 1993) reviewing the scientific publishing activities of corporations and the impact of such articles on xenobiotics, Bayer/Miles ranked number 8. To a great part it has been Alexander Scriabine's contribution that helped Bayer/Miles achieve that ranking. The papers presented at this workshop provide proof of his scientific impact, specifically in the development of calcium antagonists.

Some of the most important milestones in the development of this therapeutic concept have been presented by friends and coworkers. All of us on both sides of the Atlantic really enjoyed working with Alex and would like to thank him for all the support he has given to us.

Maybe this workshop has compensated for some of his efforts. Thanks, Alex!

Springer-Verlag and the Environment

We at Springer-Verlag firmly believe that an international science publisher has a special obligation to the environment, and our corporate policies consistently reflect this conviction.

We also expect our business partners – paper mills, printers, packaging manufacturers, etc. – to commit themselves to using environmentally friendly materials and production processes.

The paper in this book is made from low- or no-chlorine pulp and is acid free, in conformance with international standards for paper permanency.

GPSR Compliance

The European Union's (EU) General Product Safety Regulation (GPSR) is a set of rules that requires consumer products to be safe and our obligations to ensure this.

If you have any concerns about our products, you can contact us on ProductSafety@springernature.com

In case Publisher is established outside the EU, the EU authorized representative is:

Springer Nature Customer Service Center GmbH
Europaplatz 3
69115 Heidelberg, Germany

Batch number: 10704713

Printed by Printforce, the Netherlands